Studies in Social Policy and Welfare XIX
General Editor: R. A. Pinker

Health and Welfare States of Britain
An Inter-country Comparison

In the same series

I REFORMING THE WELFARE: THE POLITICS OF CHANGE IN THE PERSONAL SOCIAL SERVICES
Phoebe Hall

II UNIVERSALITY, SELECTIVITY AND EFFECTIVENESS IN SOCIAL POLICY
Bleddyn Davies

III RICHARD TITMUSS: WELFARE AND SOCIETY
David Reisman

IV RATIONING SOCIAL SERVICES: A STUDY OF RESOURCE ALLOCATION IN THE PERSONAL SOCIAL SERVICES
Ken Judge

V VIOLENCE AND THE SOCIAL SERVICES IN NORTHERN IRELAND
Edited by John Darby and Arthur Williamson

VI OLD AND COLD
Malcolm Wicks

VII THE ECONOMICS OF SOCIAL SECURITY
Leslie McClements

VIII THE WELFARE STATE IN SWEDEN
Dorothy Wilson

IX THE IDEA OF WELFARE
Robert Pinker

X PROCESS AND STRUCTURE IN HIGHER EDUCATION
Tony Becher and Maurice Kogan

XI PART-TIME SOCIAL WORK
Tony and Phoebe Hall

XII FAMILY ALLOWANCES, 1918–45: A CASE-STUDY IN SOCIAL POLICY DEVELOPMENT
John Macnicol

XIII TAXATION AND SOCIAL POLICY
Edited by Cedric Sandford, Chris Pond and Robert Walker

XIV THE RIGHT TO WELFARE AND OTHER ESSAYS
T. H. Marshall

XV DISCRETION AND WELFARE
Michael Adler and Stewart Asquith

XVI PROFESSIONAL IMPERIALISM: SOCIAL WORK IN THE THIRD WORLD
James Midgley

XVII CORPORATISM AND WELFARE: SOCIAL POLICY AND STATE INTERVENTION IN BRITAIN
Alan Cawson

XVIII THE CREATION OF THE BRITISH PERSONAL SOCIAL SERVICES 1962–1974
Joan Cooper

XIX HEALTH AND WELFARE STATES OF BRITAIN: AN INTER-COUNTRY COMPARISON
Edited by Arthur Williamson and Graham Room

XX COMMUNITY AGAINST GOVERNMENT: THE BRITISH COMMUNITY DEVELOPMENT PROJECT, 1968–1978 – A STUDY OF GOVERNMENT INCOMPETENCE
Martin Loney

Health and Welfare States of Britain

An Inter-country Comparison

Edited by ARTHUR WILLIAMSON and GRAHAM ROOM

H·E·B Heinemann Educational Books

Heinemann Educational Books
22 Bedford Square, London WC1B 3HH

LONDON EDINBURGH MELBOURNE AUCKLAND
HONG KONG SINGAPORE KUALA LUMPUR
NEW DELHI IBADAN NAIROBI JOHANNESBURG
EXETER (NH) KINGSTON PORT OF SPAIN

First published 1983

British Library Cataloguing in Publication Data

Health and welfare states of Britain an inter-country
comparison. – (Studies in social policy and welfare;
19)
1. Public welfare – Great Britain – History – 20th
century
I. Williamson, Arthur II. Room, Graham
III. Series
361'.941 HV245

ISBN 0-435-82953-X

Typeset by The Castlefield Press of Northampton
Printed by Biddles Ltd, Guildford, Surrey

Contents

Foreword

This book owes its origins to the initiative of Susan Sinclair, Senior Lecturer in Social Administration at Edinburgh University, and a past member of the Sociology and Social Administration Sub-Committee of the Social Science Research Council. As one of its series of research initiatives the Council funded a project to explore the way forward for comparative research in social policy in the United Kingdom. Arthur Williamson of the New University of Ulster was invited to convene the project and Susan Sinclair worked with him in the organisation of two workshops which were held at the London School of Economics and at the University of Edinburgh. Graham Room, Lecturer in Sociology at the University of Bath, was rapporteur for the project.

The workshop conveners received considerable encouragement and help from Professor Raymond Illsley of the University of Aberdeen. That the revised papers are now published in this volume reflects both the encouragement of Professor Bob Pinker of the London School of Economics and the endorsement by the Social Science Research Council of the Final Report of the project. The book contains a paper by Richard Berthoud which was not included in the original workshop series but which was specially commissioned for the volume.

The editors hope that the book will provide a fresh impetus for the study of contrasting patterns of policy, need and provision as between the countries and regions of the United Kingdom, a topic in which the Council has declared a continuing interest. They also hope that it may make a modest contribution to the literature concerning the development of comparative approaches to the study of social policy and administration.

Arthur Williamson
Graham Room

The Contributors

Arthur Williamson has lectured in Social Administration at the New University of Ulster since 1970. He was joint editor and contributor to *Violence and the Social Services in Northern Ireland* (1978), published in series with this volume. He is now working on a research project, funded by the SSRC, investigating trends in social and spatial mobility in higher education in Northern Ireland. Other research interests include the roles of Christian private voluntary organisations in relief and development.

Graham Room is Lecturer in Sociology at the University of Bath. He has written *The Sociology of Welfare* (Martin Robertson, 1979) and is co-author of *Europe Against Poverty* (Bedford Square Press, 1982). He has been a consultant to the EEC on its anti-poverty programmes.

Richard Berthoud is at the Policy Studies Institute where he led the UK contribution to an EEC-wide review of poverty and policy, part of the Community's anti-poverty programme. He is currently studying the operation of the reformed Supplementary Benefit scheme both in Great Britain and in Northern Ireland. His most recent books are: *Poverty and the Development of Anti-Poverty Policy in the UK* (co-author Joan C. Brown, Heinemann Educational Books, 1981) and *Fuel Debts and Hardship* (Policy Studies Institute, 1981).

Derek Birrell is Senior Lecturer in Social Administration at the New University of Ulster, where he has been since 1969. He was co-author of *Policy and Government in Northern Ireland* (Gill and Macmillan, Dublin, 1980). He has written various articles and carried out research on aspects of housing, social policy and public administration in Northern Ireland.

Chris Himsworth is a lecturer in the Department of Constitutional and Administrative Law at the University of Edinburgh. His interests include Scottish and comparative local government law and housing law.

David J. Hunter is Director of the Unit for the Study of the Elderly, Department of Community Medicine, University of Aberdeen, which is undertaking a five-year research programme on services for the elderly in Scotland. He is author of *Coping with Uncertainty: Policy and Politics in the National Health Service* (Research Studies Press/ Wiley, 1980) and several articles on health care organisation and policy.

Rudolf Klein is Professor of Social Policy and Director of the Centre for the Analysis of Social Policy at the University of Bath. His publications include *Complaints Against Doctors* (Charles Knight, 1973), *Politics of Consumer Representation* (Centre for Studies in Social Policy, 1976) and *Politics of the National Health Service* (Longman, 1983). His research interests include the comparative study of public expenditure.

Anne Ludbrook currently holds the post of Economic Adviser, Grampian Health Board, Aberdeen. She was formerly a Research Fellow at the Institute of Social and Economic Research, University of York.

Alan Maynard is Reader in Health Economics and Director of the Graduate Programme in Health Economics, University of York. He has worked as a consultant for the DHSS, WHO, OECD and the EEC.

Alan Maynard and Anne Ludbrook have published numerous papers together including 'Inequality, the National Health Service and Health Policy' in the *Journal of Public Policy* (1982, 2, 2, 97–116) and 'Thirty Years of Fruitless Endeavour? An Analysis of Government Intervention in Health Care Markets' in J. van der Gaag and M. Perlman (eds.), *Health, Economics and Health Economics* (North Holland, 1982). Alan Maynard is the author of *Health Care in the European Community* (Croom Helm, 1975) and the co-editor of *The Public Private Mix for Health* (Nuffield Provincial Hospitals Trust, 1982).

F. M. Martin is Professor of Social Administration and Head of the Department of Social Administration and Social Work, University of Glasgow. His recent publications include *Children out of Court* (with S. J. Fox and Kathleen Murray, 1981) and *The Scottish Juvenile Justice System* (with Kathleen Murray, 1982), both published by the Scottish Academic Press.

Alan Murie is a lecturer at the School for Advanced Urban Studies at the University of Bristol. His principal activities are in research and teaching on housing and housing policy. His publications include *Housing Inequality and Deprivation* (Heinemann Educational Books, 1983).

Gilbert Smith is currently Professor and Head of the Department of Social Administration at the University of Hull. Previously he held posts in the Scottish Office and at the Universities of Glasgow and Aberdeen. His publications include *Social Work and the Sociology of Organisations* (Routledge & Kegan Paul, 1979) and *Social Need: Policy, Practice and Research* (Routledge & Kegan Paul, 1980).

Gillian Stewart, formerly a social worker in inner London, is now a lecturer in the Department of Social Administration, University of Lancaster. Her main responsibilities are for undergraduate courses in social policy, the personal social services and the mass media and social policy. She has compiled the *Personal Social Services Bibliography* published by the Library Association.

John Tibbitt is a Principal Research Officer in the Central Research Unit of the Scottish Office, where he heads the Research Branch in the Social Work Services Group. He is author of *Social Workers as Mental Health Officers* (HMSO, 1978) and other papers on social services research.

1 Comparative Social Policy Research in the United Kingdom: conceptual and methodological issues*

Graham Room and *Arthur Williamson*

In the 1970s, at least four influences combined to thrust into public debate the established political relationships among the constituent nations of the United Kingdom. Entry into the European Community in 1973 put in question the traditional doctrine of the Westminster Parliament's sovereignty, while direct elections to the European Parliament in 1979 provided a direct link, bypassing Westminster, between the regions of the UK and a supranational elected body. North Sea oil, particularly following the energy crisis after 1973, fuelled Scottish nationalism and its demands for local control of Scotland's new-found wealth. The troubles in Northern Ireland spawned a multitude of proposals for reform of its constitutional relationship with the rest of the United Kingdom; indeed, closer consultation between London and Dublin lent credibility to proposals for wider constitutional reform embracing Eire also. Finally, as unemployment mounted and recession deepened in the late 1970s, the long-standing differences in the arithmetic of misery among these different nations and regions became starker and found political expression, for example, in the unprecedented division between North and South of Labour and Conservative victories in the 1979 General Election.

At a political level then, the relationship – and the differences – among these constituent nations was increasingly the subject of public debate. Of course, the differences are not confined to politics and economics but extend also to ideology and religion. Prompted by this developing debate, various social policy researchers, particularly but by no means exclusively those in Scotland and Northern Ireland, began in the later 1970s to draw attention to significant differences in social policy, social provision and social ideology existing across the British Isles. (See, for example, some of the items included in Gillian Stewart's annotated bibliography, the final chapter in this book.)

However, these, often considerable, variations have been largely

*This chapter draws heavily upon the reports prepared by Graham Room on the SSRC workshops from which this book derives.

ignored by the mainstream literature in the subject. Most textbooks used on undergraduate courses give scant attention to variations from the English model of service provision and delivery, assuming implicitly that 'English' equals 'British'. This might be explained in structural terms, having regard to the distribution of university departments of social administration and, consequently, to the main markets for textbooks. But the assumptions that underlie this limited view are not confined to teachers of social administration and their students. Administrators, policy-makers and advisers in many social service fields often appear unaware of the very great variations which exist in legislation, structures, practices, social conditions and political and religio-cultural assumptions between the different parts of the United Kingdom (and between the regions of England and the metropolis). Moreover, there is accumulating evidence that those with responsibility for formulating social policy in Scotland and in Northern Ireland (particularly under direct rule) may often follow political guidance or fashion which has more relevance to conditions in the south of England than to those areas for which they have direct responsibility.

It is, of course, true that the periphery can, and does, influence the centre. One striking illustration of this is found with reference to some of the quite remarkable social innovations of English administrators in nineteenth-century Ireland, for instance in the field of provision for the mentally ill, and in prison administration, where experimental models were developed which were to have an impact on the planning of social policy in England.[1] Northern Ireland now has an integrated structure for the administration and delivery of health and personal social services introduced in 1973 under the direct rule administration (discussed by Derek Birrell and Arthur Williamson in Chapter 8). Perhaps the province is being used once again as a test-bed for social policy innovation for the mainland? Certainly it would be surprising if some of the English junior ministers charged with the responsibility for managing services there did not, on their return to Westminster, carry with them principles and ideas tempered in the crucible of Ulster.

To repeat, however, this potentially valuable ground for research has largely been neglected by the mainstream literature. This is puzzling at a time when British academics are giving increasing attention to international comparative social policy research. There is a 'missing middle' between the present focus of comparative social policy research on international questions on the one hand and a growing number of useful studies of local variations on the other.

This contrasts to some other academic disciplines where comparative studies have been in vogue for some time. In education for example, comparative studies are at least in their adolescence although even there

Robert Bell and Nigel Grant in their *Patterns of Education in the British Isles* caution that comparative educationalists 'with few exceptions have not paid much attention to the educational and cultural pluralism of their own islands'.[2]

Two questions are raised by this neglect of variety and of differences in levels of social provision, need, administrative structures, legislation and political ideology. First, what types of comparative study might most usefully concern themselves with these intra-UK variations? Secondly, how may we account for the relative neglect to date? These questions provide the focus for the discussion that follows and also for the contributions of Rudolf Klein and Fred Martin in Part One of this book.

No collection can hope by itself to fill this 'missing middle'. In an effort to demonstrate the usefulness of comparative policy studies in one area and to narrow the book's field of vision, the arena chosen for Part Two is the health and personal social services. Nevertheless, in Part Three, contributions appear which deal with other areas of social policy, and illustrate how the detailed treatment of differences may be applied in other areas of social provision and, in the case of housing, demonstrate that intra-Britain comparative studies have recently advanced to a level of considerable importance to policy-makers. Later in this chapter some of the principal points to emerge from these empirical chapters will be drawn together.

Comparison in social policy research[3]

The value of comparative studies

Durkheim argued that 'comparative sociology is not a particular branch of sociology; it is sociology itself'.[4] Some have seen comparative study as a means of approximating to – or rather, perhaps, substituting for – the experimental method of the natural sciences. With regard to policy studies, Gilbert Smith argues in Chapter 7 of this volume that comparative analysis provides an alternative approach to the use of time-series data. The Seebohm reform of personal social service structures in England, for example, did not find a counterpart in Scotland. Comparisons across the border can help to illuminate some aspects of the consequences of reform in England. Again, comparative studies can be employed to curb misplaced generalisation: certainly many of the contributors to this volume aim to challenge the assumptions of homogeneity which they see policy-makers and researchers as too prone to make.

The logic of comparative studies

Although social researchers and policy-makers alike have tended often to overlook variations in policy and services among the constituent nations of the UK, these variations are, on closer inspection, legion. Some of our contributors call for more detailed description of these differences, as the necessary – if theoretically unpretentious – precondition for systematic research. Of these, some see such efforts as filling a major gap in the data currently available; others seem, in effect, to take inspiration from the biological sciences, arguing that the first steps to developing a taxonomy are observation, description and classification of individual differences.

Nevertheless, it is also true that many aspects of policy and services are similar. This is an advantage when contrasted with international comparative studies because it means that some important variables can be 'held constant', while the other elements are explored in some detail. Inspection of these differences in ideology, policy and services can therefore generate a multitude of research questions. In several of the contributions to this volume, the authors offer 'research agendas' of this sort. However, this offers at once too much and too little: too much, because it provides a multitude of topics, each suitable for a doctoral thesis; too little, because it fails to suggest any principle for selecting the variations most deserving of attention. More fundamentally, however, it can be argued that simple *inspection* of these variations cannot of itself generate the *questions* without which no enquiry can begin.

Rather, it is first necessary to define the questions to be researched: only then can the particular geographical and institutional focus of the research be chosen. 'If the right questions can be identified, superfluous description is avoided and appropriate departure points for analysis can be located.'[5] Rudolf Klein suggests that questions may be pitched at the macro level, concerned with explaining 'the evolution or the behaviour of the system as a whole', in which case the researcher will best select countries that differ in terms of their political and social ideologies, macro organisation and institutions. At the opposite extreme, questions may be pitched at the micro level, concerned with explaining how a specific policy works in different contexts or, alternatively, how different policies work in broadly the same context; here the researcher will choose countries that are broadly similar in terms of their economic development, social organisation and political ideology (see Chapter 2 of this volume).

If comparisons among the constituent nations of the United Kingdom are to be useful, therefore, it will most often be in relation to questions pitched at this micro level (see also Chapter 3 of this work). Even so, the researcher will not in general find the experience of other countries irrelevant to even those micro level questions most susceptible to treatment by intra-UK comparisons; it will often be convenience alone which justifies such a restriction of his attention.

How are the questions themselves to be chosen? As in all social policy research, the choice of a 'good' question must be made in terms of its theoretical interest and its policy relevance, whether the questions are pitched at the micro or macro level. The contributors to Parts Two and Three of this book tend to justify their particular interests on these two counts. At the same time, however – and again, as in all good social policy research – this leads them also to reflect critically not only upon the conventional sets of theoretical questions which they have inherited as members of a research community, but also upon the parameters within which policy-makers frame *their* questions. They point, for example, to the readiness of central government policy-makers to assume both homogeneity across the UK in their field of action and the general relevance of the English model of policy provision. One important purpose of their intra-UK comparative research is to contest these assumptions and to illuminate the social, economic and political variations that mould the differential operation of central government policies.

The content of comparative studies

Granted the potential interest and value of intra-UK comparative studies, why focus upon the constituent *nations*? One justification might be that here is an obvious and important gap in contemporary social policy studies. However, some of the contributors to this book, notably Murie (Chapter 10), prefer to consider different *regions*, each defined in terms of its distinctive pattern of social provision. Alan Murie reviews the housing literature over recent decades and points to the preoccupation with administrative arrangements at a local authority level, which he considers as at best out of fashion and at worst misplaced. He argues that the appropriate basis on which to consider housing is the regional one and that this takes account of economic realities without which housing cannot be considered in a holistic fashion. Even here, however, a concern with the national level is not inappropriate since, at least in the case of Northern Ireland, separate legislation and, until the early 1970s, different sets of assumptions concerning the role of public housing, led to very great differences in policy and provision as compared with Great Britain.

Certainly interregional studies are an important focus for intra-UK comparative research. Indeed, Murie's approach, considering housing provision as the developing response to uneven patterns of economic and industrial development, provides a further rationale for intra-UK comparative studies: for the regions of the UK have closely interrelated economic histories and form parts of a coherently developing whole. At the same time, however, Murie does not see administrative and legislative provisions as merely a response to the development of the capitalist economy; instead he invites a more sophisticated exploration and appreciation of their mutual interaction.

The dearth of intra-UK comparative studies

Why have intra-UK comparative studies been relatively neglected? Most of our contributors, most obviously Gilbert Smith, at least touch on this question and between them they suggest four complementary explanations. First, much applied social policy research is undertaken on behalf of central government policy-makers and tends to adopt their assumption of homogeneity across the United Kingdom. Indeed, central government appears often to subscribe to the maxim that comparisons are invidious and is interested in comparisons only when they aid debate over resource allocation, for example.[6]

Secondly, social researchers who have pioneered comparative studies have tended to look beyond these islands for their comparisons. In part this is because many have been interested in macro level differences in social policies and social stystems. It is also, however, a response to the concerns of central government and its critics, who eagerly look to the social policies of central governments elsewhere in justification – or criticism – of domestic policies. (In general, therefore, and perhaps necessarily, the questions that are posed even at the macro level tend to be rooted in the domestic research and policy agenda.)

Thirdly, the question of *competence* takes a particularly stark form in the case of intra-UK comparisons. To start with, few international comparative researchers can claim to be equally familiar with all the different regions or countries they are comparing. In general, however, their readership is drawn from the researcher's 'home ground' and is even less familiar than he is with the other countries under discussion. Intra-UK studies allow no such self-protection, however, and for many researchers the challenge to professional self-esteem is, perhaps, too great. So too, those engaged in comparative intra-UK studies cannot excuse their efforts by reference to the linguistic barriers they have encountered and they must expect a less indulgent readership.

Finally, many of the existing sources of data are ill-suited to intra-UK comparative studies. As Richard Berthoud notes, official statistics often appear to be arbitrary in regard to 'how many of the countries will be included at all, how many will be combined for summary purposes, how many will be identifiable in detailed analysis'. Rose and McAllister have recently attempted to bring some order to this situation,[7] but in the field of social policy at least, much remains to be done.

Health and personal social services

The essays in Part Two of this book consider aspects of the health and personal social services. Chris Himsworth provides a comparative analysis of the legislative provisions in health and the personal social services. His paper considers not only the functions, responsibilities and composition of the various statutory authorities, but also the formal relationships between different levels of authority and the provisions for consultation with the public and for liaison between health and personal social services. This paper provides essential background to those that follow.

The next two papers are concerned with the health services in different parts of the United Kingdom. David Hunter focuses upon the different patterns of health service reorganisation undertaken over the 1970s and the resulting administrative and institutional arrangements. The themes of the reorganisation that he uses to structure his discussion are threefold: integration, management and planning. Within each, he combines examination of the formal organisational arrangements and the way these operate in practice. His paper then raises, if it does not answer, various further questions in relation to policy implementation and outcomes: for example, the part played by the 'issue networks' of service professionals, local opinion leaders and organised lobbies.

Alan Maynard and Anne Ludbrook look at variations in health care resources. More specifically, they examine the construction and application of the various resource allocation formulae that health policy-makers have developed in recent years – the RAWP (Resource Allocation Working Party) formula in England and analogous formulae in Wales (SCRAW), Scotland (SHARE) and Northern Ireland (PARR). What these authors have elsewhere[8] attempted is to apply one of these formulae to the total health budgets of the four constituent nations: the results suggest that Scotland and Northern Ireland are relatively well-treated (although weaknesses in the raw data again point to the difficulties of providing definitive comparisons of this kind). A less ambitious follow-up study might be to examine how far the differences in the way these various formulae were constructed might derive from the differences in the social, political and institutional contexts of the different nations, or how far they reflect policy-makers' efforts to learn from – and improve upon – the efforts of their counterparts elsewhere.

Gilbert Smith's paper has a dual focus. He examines the organisation of social work and juvenile justice – both areas of important legal change and administrative reorganisation since the early 1970s – and the differences apparent between Scotland and England. He points to the lack of systematic research in these fields, within each country as well as between them, and offers suggestions as to fruitful lines of enquiry. Secondly, he goes on to examine the institutional *barriers* that have inhibited intra-UK comparative studies in these fields; his comments have provided the basis for much of what was said in the previous section of this chapter.

Part Two of this book is completed with the contributions on the relationship between the health and personal social services. Derek Birrell and Arthur Williamson write about Northern Ireland, the only part of the United Kingdom to have so far integrated health and personal social services into one management and planning structure. They consider why Northern Ireland has followed this distinctive pattern of development and provide a comprehensive review of the experience of operating the integrated structure for the last ten years culminating in the restructuring exercise which followed from the *Report* of the Royal Commission on the National Health Service.

As John Tibbett observes, throughout the UK reorganisation of these services since 1970 has had as a central aim their more effective planning and collaboration. He exploits various sociological perspectives to analyse the organisational interface between the two services: an interface which differs significantly as between the different nations of the United Kingdom. He is equally concerned with their strategic planning and their day-to-day collaboration. He analyses the strategies of interaction that professionals in the two services follow in order to promote their respective interests.

Although directing their attention to the health and personal social services, all these essays go beyond the formal organisational provisions (except of course for Chris Himsworth, who aims to provide the legislative background to these comparisons). They examine the tensions and conflicts between different levels of government and administration and the way in which power is exercised within the different administrative frameworks in different parts of the UK. They point to the importance of professional and consumer attitudes in moulding service provisions and highlight these issues as areas for worthwhile comparative study and to the different sorts of 'issue network' (including not least the relationships between the research and policy-making communities) that may exist in different parts of the UK, as a variable influencing policy implementation.

Part Three ventures into other areas of social policy, in order to demonstrate that these intra-UK comparisons are by no means of interest only in respect of health and the personal social services and to explore the extent to which a comparative approach already has been developed. As noted earlier Alan Murie considers the relationship between housing provision and uneven patterns of economic and industrial development in different regions. His approach is strongly historical and it directs attention to regions defined in terms of their industrial histories rather than to the administratively separate nations of the United Kingdom. He suggests that future intra-UK studies must consider the interaction between the different policy-making and administrative frameworks of the different *nations* on the one hand and the patterns of *regional* economic development on the other, in moulding the social needs and service provisions of different areas.

Finally, Richard Berthoud investigates intra-UK variations in low incomes and the effectiveness of social security and other public programmes in redressing these imbalances. In the course of his essay, he examines in some detail the pitfalls to obtaining reliable data on the four nations of the UK in a form which will allow meaningful comparisons to be made.

Prospects for intra-UK comparative studies

Whereas there has, as yet, been a dearth of intra-UK comparative studies it is possible to observe a number of trends which make it likely that this subject will receive more attention in the fairly near future. During the 1970s social administration became increasingly spatial in its approach, reflecting to some degree research findings on the distribution of poverty and morbidity.[9] Geographical variations in unemployment and in the distribution of health service resources have also received more attention and research. The Labour administration of Harold Wilson set up the Resource Allocation Working Party and for the first time a thoroughgoing attempt was made to allocate resources between and within regions on the basis of demonstrable need. Publications such as the Black Report on Health Inequalities (1980)[10] focused attention on regional disparities with regard to need. Further, new concern with the themes of social justice and citizenship during the 1970s has led to increasing attention being paid to geographical, as well as social, inequities. Julia Parker's *Social Policy and Citizenship* (1975) helped bring some of these questions into prominence for social administrators.[11]

Of course, intra-UK comparative studies will continue to face the institutional obstacles discussed earlier in this chapter. Current debates over the funding and orientation of social science research make it more, not less, likely that central government interests will tend to prevail in setting the questions to be investigated. Recent restrictions on the government's statistical services hardly make this a propitious moment to press for more systematic and adequate data on variations among the component parts of the United Kingdom.

Nevertheless, the Social Science Research Council workshops from which this book originated have provided a valuable stimulus to intra-UK research into comparative social policy questions. They served to illustrate the importance of the comparative dimension, to bring into the open some of the questions and problems which have tended to inhibit the development of the subject and, further, to focus attention on a growing number of studies produced by researchers in different disciplines, many of whom have been working in virtual isolation. We hope that publication of this volume will encourage a still wider interest among social policy researchers and an increased awareness both of the opportunities and of the value of comparative social policy research.

Notes

1. Oliver MacDonagh develops this thesis in his *Ireland*, Prentice-Hall 1968, p. 23 and quotes W. L. Burn who observed that nineteenth century Ireland formed a 'social laboratory. . . . The most conventional of Englishmen were willing to experiment in Ireland on lines which they were not prepared to contemplate or tolerate at home'. (W. L. Burn, 'Free Trade in Land: An aspect of the Irish Question', *Transactions of the Royal Historical Society*, 4th ser., Vol. XXXI, p. 68).
2. London: Geo. Allen and Unwin, 1977, p. 13.
3. This section is indebted to the paper 'Approaches to comparison in Social Policy' which Joan Higgins contributed to the first of the Social Science Research Council workshops on comparative social policy research from which this book originated.
4. *Rules of Sociological Method*, New York: Free Press, 1938, p. 139, quoted and discussed in Joan Higgins, *States of Welfare*, London: Martin Robertson, 1981, p. 13.
5. Higgins, *op. cit.*, p. 2; see also Higgins, 1981.
6. See, for example, the closing remarks in Martin's essay (Chapter 3 of this volume).
7. R. Rose and J. McAllister, *United Kingdom Facts*, London: Macmillan, 1982.
8. 'Applying Resource Allocation Formulae to Constituent Parts of the United Kingdom', *Lancet*, 1980, Vol. i, pp. 85–8.
9. See for example 'Social Policy goes Spatial', in David Donnison with Paul Soto, *The Good City: a study of urban development and policy in Britain*, London: Heinemann Educational Books, 1980.
10. Department of Health and Social Security, *Inequalities in Health: Report of a Research Working Group*, (The Black Report), 1980.
11. London: Macmillan, 1975.

PART ONE
Principles of Comparative Research

2 Strategies for Comparative Social Policy Research

Rudolf Klein

Why should we be interested in comparing social policies across nations? Broadly speaking, there would appear to be two quite different reasons for indulging in this exercise – each of which would seem to require a rather different research strategy.

First, there is what might be called *policy learning.*[1] That is, we look at the social policies of other countries in order to derive lessons or models which can be applied at home. This approach has a long history. The example of Bismarck's legislation was much studied and debated before the introduction of Lloyd George's 1911 insurance reforms.[2] Royal Commissions and Committees of Inquiry regularly draw on the experience of other countries: see, for instance, the Finer Report.[3] Similarly, academics may use other countries heuristically: as laboratories where particular ideas are being tested. Given the problems of testing social policies experimentally, using the experience of other countries in this way is particularly attractive.

Second, there is what might be called *policy understanding*. Here the emphasis is not so much on learning as on explanation. For example, if we are to achieve an understanding of the factors which shape the evolution of a social security system, it is unlikely that we can do so by looking at one country in isolation. Are the key variables the level of industrialisation and the political mobilisation of the working class? The history of Britain, examined in isolation, might suggest that they are. But comparative studies indicate otherwise.[4] Similarly, it has been argued that in Britain the power of the medical profession rests on its access to Whitehall,[5] while comparative studies show that the nature of that power is largely independent of the precise relationship between doctors and bureaucracy.[6] In short, comparative studies may be essential if misleading conclusions are not to be drawn from what are single case studies in the making, or evolution, of social policy.

The research strategies associated with these two approaches would to judge from the literature, seem to be: First, a micro strategy (or single issue approach) in 'most similar' countries, keeping numbers down. That is, the prime concern is not with the nature of the social policy *system*, since it is implausible to assume that a total system can be transplanted from one country to another, but a discrete area of policy. In turn, this means comparing countries that are judged to be roughly similar in terms of economic development, social organisation and political ideology. For if the focus of concern is the transplantability of ideas or models, then it is clearly essential that the two environments should not be too different (although in practice the literature in this area tends to make very rough and ready assumptions about which countries can sensibly be compared, and the discussion of what are judged to be the crucial dimensions of similarity is rarely explicit). Lastly, the learning or laboratory approach usually means limiting the number of cases studied: the greater the number of cases, the greater also the risk of noise in the machine – of dissimilarities creeping in – so invalidating the whole point of the exercise.

Second, a macro strategy (or systems approach) in 'most different' countries, using large numbers. In this approach the focus of interest are the factors that help to explain either the evolution or the behaviour of the *system* as a whole. The nature of the analysis therefore positively requires differences in the economic development, social organisation or political ideology of the countries being examined (for it is obviously impossible to test the significance of a specific factor if it is common to all the cases being examined). Large numbers, in as far as they allow a statistical analysis of the factors concerned, are an additional advantage. But as with the micro strategy, the criteria for admitting specific cases, while excluding others, are often somewhat fudged: the availability of data often appears to be the determining factor. The bias of these studies is towards concentrating on those variables – e.g. levels of expenditure – that can be quantified.

Both the intellectual approaches and the research strategies tend to have a disciplinary bias. The policy learning approach, with its micro-strategy of research, tends to be favoured by social policy specialists: indeed at times the interest in foreign experience seems to derive mainly from anxiety to get new polemical ammunition. The policy understanding approach, with its macro strategy of research, tends to be favoured more by political scientists and sociologists. The strength of the former lies in its ability to convey the 'texture' of social policies: what these actually mean to the people involved. Its weakness derives from the failure to place individual policies in the wider economic, social and administrative context. In contrast, the strength of the latter lies in its potential capacity to handle political, economic and social variables. But its weakness derives from its frequent inability to cope with the fine print of social policy, and its overreliance on what are often rough and ready statistical indicators.

In drawing this contrast, I have obviously dichotomised the literature somewhat brutally. There are a number of studies – and these are usually the best – which do not fall neatly into my two categories.[7] For example, my categorisation does not easily accommodate the broad-brush descriptive comparison of welfare systems taken as a whole. However, the point of my deliberately over-simple analysis of the literature is to argue that, in thinking about research strategies for comparative studies, we should attempt to combine the two approaches. In other words, we should use specific issues as 'tracers' in order to see how different systems operate: how the same issue fares, in other words, when processed by a different 'issue-machine'.[8]

The implications of this approach are twofold. First, that the issues chosen as 'tracers' should be picked not just because they are judged to be interesting in a general sort of way but because they are relevant to crucial questions in social policy. In other words, we need an analytic – as distinct from a merely descriptive – categorisation of issues. For example, it is often argued that social policy is primarily about redistribution.[9] This might suggest that analytically crucial issues are those involving the redistribution of either power or resources (and the two, of course, often go hand in hand). But if it is argued that social policy cannot be summed up quite so neatly – which would be my own view – then perhaps we should extend our search for issues which would serve as analytic tin-openers. For instance, we might choose issues that test the reactions of different systems to environmental shocks: their capacity, as it were, to react to – or to handle – new developments, such as economic recession or technological change. Further, we might choose issues that help us to ask questions about the power structure of different systems: directing attention at those policy areas which allow us to examine the influence of service providers (professional and others) in different systems. Again, we might choose issues that permit us to compare the relative 'rationality' of different systems by asking how far their allocation of resources – or policy priorities – conform to the general societal 'needs' by looking at the match (or lack of it) between what is done, perceived needs and any objective social indicators that we may be able to find. The list is illustrative, not exhaustive: the main point is to underline the need for clarity in choosing the issues chosen as 'tracers'.

Turning to the systems, it is again crucial to be clear as to what are the relevant variables (if only to know whether or not, in choosing the countries to compare, certain variables are being kept constant). Again, the object of this exercise is not to compile an exhaustive list of variables. But certain clusters are conventionally used in the literature and can be identified without difficulty. There are economic variables: for example the level of national income. There are political variables: the hegemonic ideology, the pattern of party support. There are organisational variables:

the relationship between local and central government, the administrative structure of particular services. Lastly, there are what might be called population variables: it cannot be assumed that the particular problem being addressed by social policy-makers is necessarily comparable in scale or complexity even if it (misleadingly) comes under the same label – the nature of poverty is not the same in a developed and in an under-developed country, in highly industrialised and in predominantly agricultural societies, in a country where low income is predominantly associated with black skins and in a country where it is racially neutral.

All this is not to suggest that, in choosing our strategies for comparative research, we are yet in a position to devise a methodology which can cope with all these variables – although some ingenious and heroic attempts to do so have been made.[10] It is, however, to suggest that any strategy must make an *explicit* judgement about why particular countries are being compared – in what respects they are 'most similar' or 'most different' – and what the object of the whole exercise is: whether it is simply to gain an understanding of how individual national models of welfare operate or whether it is to try to draw some general conclusions about the interaction between such models and the societal environments, or systems, of which they are part.

A further distinction should perhaps be drawn in analysing the strategies available for comparative research. On the one hand there are those studies which primarily seek to *describe* the institutions and provisions of the Welfare State (an unfortunate label to the extent that it tends to divert attention from the role of public policies in shaping the private provision of welfare)– an important ground-clearing exercise in its own right. On the other hand, there are those studies that seek to *evaluate* those institutions and provisions and are in effect looking for a 'best buy' model – and thus move into the boggy territory of trying to assess the effect of policies (which immediately raises questions about the criteria to be used and difficulties about assessing the nature of the problems being addressed, and to what extent these are comparable in the first place). Again, this categorisation is over-simple: it excludes the important category of studies which analyse the *process* of policy-making and implementation.[11] However, the main point remains: comparative studies of social policy are not homogeneous – and although the various categories are not mutually exclusive, it may be helpful to keep these distinctions in mind when discussing future research strategy.

The case of England, Scotland and Northern Ireland

In the light of what has been said above, England, Scotland and Northern

Ireland would seem to be natural candidates for comparative studies. Studying these three countries would, on the face of it, appear to control for a large number of systems variables. Such a strategy would therefore seem to have the advantage of allowing a strictly limited number of differences to be studied: specifically, differences in the *organisational* structure of services. (The union of health and personal social services in Northern Ireland; the distribution of responsibilities within the NHS in Scotland.)

All three countries are roughly at the same level of economic development, despite some differences in per capita income. All three governments, additionally, come under the same system of parliamentary government. Even the basic legislative framework of the main social services concerned is the same; the methods of financing them and the levels of service provider remuneration are common to them all. Lastly, and not unimportantly, all three collect statistics on a roughly comparable basis. But it is perhaps equally important to stress the systems differences. Most obviously, the three countries are enormously disparate in terms of population (England, 46,500,000; Scotland, 5,200,000; Northern Ireland, 1,500,000). This raises an immediate problem. If we find any differences in the effectiveness of a particular service, should we attribute this to the particular structural characteristics of the organisation concerned, or to problems raised or opportunities created by large or small size? To be able to answer such a question, we should perhaps have to compare not just these three countries but a matched sample of countries of similar size. For example, we might consider comparing Scotland not just with England but also with Denmark or Finland, and Northern Ireland with Luxembourg.

Alternatively, this point may suggest that in comparative studies attention should be paid to identifying and analysing social policy networks: i.e. that we should study the nature of the contacts and relationships between those involved in social policy at all levels and all stages in the process – from policy formation to implementation. A fairly obvious hypothesis to develop is that the nature of these networks will differ depending on the size of the country involved, and that the smaller the country the greater will be the ability to rely on informal methods. It might further be argued that the problems of policy implementation should have an inverse relationship to size: the smaller the country, the more will those who implement policy have been involved in the process of policy formulation, with the result that there should be a greater congruence between the two.

Again, the similarities in the political systems are deceptive. All three countries have the same system of parliamentary elections; all three come under the legislative umbrella of Westminster. But Northern Ireland is characterised by religious cleavages, the absence of normal politics at the local level, and the lack of the kind of over-arching consensus about fundamentals which normally constrains conflicts.[12] Scotland is characterised by the presence of a strong separatist/federalist movement. Consequently one of the factors which has to be examined is the possibility (to put it with extreme caution) that Scotland may have the advantage when it comes to resource distribution: that the politics of social policy may reflect the desire of the two national parties to whip the carpet from under the feet of the nationalist. Certainly, as Table 2.1 shows, Scotland does considerably better than England in getting resources for the health and personal social services – although Northern Ireland does even better.

Table 2.1 Per capita spending on the health and personal social services (£, 1978 survey prices)

England	148
Scotland	181
N. Ireland	187

Source: *The Government's Expenditure Plans 1979/80 to 1982/83*, London: HMSO, 1979, Cmnd 7439.

This would seem to suggest that it might be fruitful to compare Scotland and Northern Ireland with other countries where there are either strong separatist movements or internal cleavages along religious or ethnic lines. Thus in the case of Scotland it might be revealing to compare its experience with that of, say, Quebec: i.e. making the existence of separatist movement the criterion of selection for comparison. Similarly, in the case of Northern Ireland it might be interesting to compare its experience with that of, for example, Belgium: i.e. making the existence of distributional conflict along ethnic/religious lines the criterion of selection for comparison.

There are also differences in the population characteristics of the three countries which suggest that the nature of the social policy problems being addressed cannot be assumed to be identical. As Table 2.2 shows the age structure of the population differs considerably. Taking the two groups, the young and the old, that are most relevant for the health and personal social services (in that they account for a disportionate amount of the consumption), England is the mirror image of Northern Ireland with a higher proportion of the elderly and a lower proportion of the young, although whether the differences are significant enough to affect policy is a question which requires further investigation. Similarly, as Table 2.3 shows, using some of the conventional indicators of the state of a population's health – standardised mortality ratios

Table 2.2 Population structure 1977

	% of population age 0–14	*% of population aged 65+*
England	22.2	14.4
Scotland	23.1	13.5
Northern Ireland	26.7	13.3

Source: *Social Trends No. 9*, London: HMSO, 1978.

(SMRs) and infant mortality – England appears to have a considerably healthier population than the other two countries (which might, in turn, suggest that – to return to Table 2.1 – Scotland and Northern Ireland get an appropriate share of resources when their needs are taken into account, although, as the RAWP debate has demonstrated,[13] there are considerable problems about basing criteria of resource allocation equity on the available indicators). The indicators are, however, ambiguous in their implications for social policy.

Table 2.3 Indicators of health, 1976

	Standardised mortality ratios		*Infant mortality*
	M	*F*	*(per 1000 births)*
England	100	100	14.3
Scotland	114	111	14.8
Northern Ireland	114	117	18.3

Source: *On the State of the Public Health, 1977*, HMSO 1978. (Note that the figures for England include those for Wales.)

Poor performance on the conventional health indicators may be taken to mean either that more money should be spent on health or, given the evidence, that expenditure on health care does not appear to be linked to health status,[14] that more money should be spent in other areas of social policy – e.g. nutrition, housing or income maintenance.

In turn, this may suggest the importance in comparative research of examining the policy instruments used in different systems in order to deal with a particular problem – which might well be perceived as a health care issue in one country, while it might be defined as an income maintenance issue in another. Although the next and final section of this paper deals specifically with the health and personal social services, it is important to stress the dangers of an approach that takes its parameters from the existing administrative arrangements: given the scope for substitution as between different social services (for example help to the aged may, at the margins at least, take the form either of cash or of services), any comparative analysis of particular services must first ask itself about the extent to which their role and function is defined in the same way. The differential perception and definition of problems is, in itself, an important area of comparative studies.

The case of the health and personal social services

Comparative studies of health care are – in contrast to the extremely sparse and predominantly descriptive literature on personal social services – reasonably plentiful.[15] Two strands are particularly worth distinguishing. There is what might be called the 'top-down' approach: this takes as its starting-point the concerns of those running the services – such issues as the structure of services, the distribution of manpower and other resources, problems of finance, and so on.[16] There is also the 'bottom-up' approach: this is population-based, and asks questions about access in relationship to need (in so far as this controversial concept can be operationalised). The second approach has – for reasons of cost, no doubt – only produced one major study,[17] and only one attempt has been made to combine the two approaches.[18]

The 'top-down', or macro, approach has produced some interesting literature. It is particularly appropriate, of course, when testing general theories of social policy development: in particular, theories of convergence (where the finding is that different systems, under pressure of financial constraints, tend to adopt very similar strategies of resource distribution). Similarly, this approach allows – using the learning model of comparative research – the implications of using different policy instruments in similar systems to be examined: note, for example, the work on the comparative success of the United States and Canada in containing 'medical inflation'.[19] Again, using this methodology, it is possible to compare the distribution of doctors in different countries, in order to see whether maldistribution is a function of the specific organisation or particular health care systems or whether it reflects a more general problem of persuading doctors to go to unpopular or unattractive places: the answer would seem to be the latter – since even the Soviet Union, with its regimented labour force, has its under-doctored regions.[20]

The 'bottom-up' approach has produced a much more sparse literature, because there is not much ready-made population-based data and new data, as already noted, is expensive to generate. The six-country WHO study cited above is the most ambitious attempt yet. It generated survey data not only about the use of health services but also about the population's state of health. However, the six countries appear to have been chosen simply because of the availability of funds: no particular rationale for choosing these six, as distinct from others, is evident. Moreover, the analysis of the health care systems – let alone of the environmental social and political systems – is inadequate. And although the six countries offered an opportunity for grouping on the 'most similar' and 'most different' principle no such attempt was made. In contrast, Anderson's comparative study of the United States, Sweden and England is conceptually much more sophisticated – and attempts to draw together population-based data and an analysis of the systems – but it suffers from the famine of information about use and access that was available to him at the time of writing.

Turning to the specific case of England, Scotland and Northern Ireland, the trouble appears to be that they are too similar. What at first sight seems to be so inviting – the fact that they share the same organisational characteristics – turns out, on closer inspection, to pose real difficulties for comparative research. Quite clearly, their experience is irrelevant for many of the standard and major concerns of comparative research in the field of health care that have been outlined above. They have converged already in most respects – finance and basic organisational structure. If, for example, there are differences in their ability to achieve a good distribution of doctors, it would be difficult to attribute this to organisational variables (which to judge from the international literature are not crucial anyway) since the success may be attributable to cultural differences – for example the fact that Scots like to live in Scotland.

Even where there are important differences – as in the combination of health and personal social services in Northern Ireland under the same authorities – there are problems of analysis, particularly when taking the 'top-down' approach. What conceptual tools have we got at our disposal for analysing the difference that such an arrangement makes? And how – to return to an earlier point – can we be sure that any differences do not simply reflect the circumstances of a country which is only marginally larger than the Birmingham conurbation? (Perhaps this comparison offers us a clue: it may be that any inquiry should be into inter-service resource planning not between England and Northern Ireland, but between Northern Ireland and a large city region divided between a variety of health authorities and PSS Departments.) Certainly the one attempt that has been made to try to answer the question of whether the Northern Irish system offers any advantages over a split-system proved singularly unconvincing: it failed to define any clear criteria for evaluating success or failure and relied on the views of those working in the services concerned.[21] Given that the main point of any research in this area would be to test a particular organisational model – i.e. the Northern Irish – and that, consequently, we are talking about evaluative research, it would seem essential to be quite clear about the criteria to be used for any such exercise – and, equally important, to be sure that we are able to isolate the organisational variables from the other environmental factors that have been discussed.

Given these kinds of difficulties, even in the one self-evident case where there are significant organisational differences, one possible strategy may be to treat the organisational structures of the three countries as 'black boxes'. Instead of devoting research energies to a description of the differences in organisational structure (or legislative provision), we could start with the question of whether in practice these matter. That is, we could take specific issues and see how, if at all, the three countries differ in the way they handle them: whether at the policy making or policy implementation stage. In other words, I am suggesting that the strategy should be to start by examining the behaviour of the three systems, rather than beginning with detailed organisational analysis. If, then, it appears that there is a difference in outcome or effect, it will be possible to work backward in seeking the explanation (which, to repeat, cannot be assumed to derive exclusively from the nature of the health or personal social service systems).

What issues could usefully be employed as 'tracers' in such a strategy? To take the example, already discussed, of the relationship between the health and personal social services, one approach might be to see whether the Northern Irish system is more successful in implementing government policies for allocating resources for the elderly and the mentally ill and handicapped to the community care sector: in other words, we could analyse the actual pattern of resource allocation. It might also be possible to test the ability of the three systems to respond 'rationally' to the problems with which they have to deal: to see whether Scotland and Northern Ireland, which have a higher rate of infant mortality than England, also devote a higher proportion of their resources to maternal care. Again, moving to the implementation of policy and the role of professional service providers, the pattern of NHS abortions might be used as a tracer: to what extent have the three countries been able to provide access to abortion facilities following the change in legislation?

Adopting a 'bottom-up' approach would suggest examining the performance of the health and personal social services in the three countries as it affects the population. For example, we might seek to develop a comparative indicator of health care access: i.e. ask whether, for any given condition, the chances of getting treatment (and if so, what kind of treatment at what level of intensity) are the same in the three countries.[22] Similarly, in the case of the personal social services, we might ask what the chances of an elderly person – with specified normative needs – are of getting particular forms of help.[23] Similarly, we might seek to develop a comparative indicator of consumer assessments of the services provided, despite the notorious problems involved. These derive from the fact that what people get tends to influence what people expect. However, it could be argued that if a particular social service manages to satisfy its clients – even though standards, on professional criteria, are low – then this in itself is a sign of success: expectations-engineering is an important aspect of social policy.

The difficulty about the 'bottom-up' approach is the scarcity of existing data, and the expense of collecting new data. For example, the General Household Survey provides information about both self-reported morbidity and the use of health services – for England, Scotland and Wales, but not for Northern Ireland. And although various attempts[24] have been made to derive an access ratio from the GHS – by looking at the relationship between the morbidity and the use data – there are reasons for scepticism as to whether the data can support such analyses.[25]

Thus Table 2.4 would suggest that Scotland offers a greater degree of access to GP services for any given amount of illness (whether short or long-term) than England – which is consistent with the fact that Scotland also gets more per capita resources. However this is to assume

Table 2.4 Indicators of morbidity and use of health services

	Limiting long-standing illness		*Restricted activity*		*GP consultation rates per year*	
	M	*F*	*M*	*F*	*M*	*F*
England	100	100	100	100	3.2	4.3
Scotland	95	87	93	82	3.7	4.8
Wales	138	111	100	122	4.2	5.2

Source: *The General Household Survey, 1972*, London: HMSO, 1974.

that self-reported morbidity data is independent of social and cultural factors, which it patently is not: hence perhaps the curious contrast between the evidence of Table 2.3, which shows that Scotland's population is less healthy than that of England using SMRs as an indicator, and that of Table 2.4, which shows precisely the reverse using self-reported morbidity as an indicator. In any case, this data about the use of GP services would have to be complemented with data about use of hospital services before any conclusions could be drawn about the performance of the health care system as a whole, since one of the issues in comparative health care research is precisely the extent to which different systems treat patients in the ambulatory, as distinct from the institutional, sector.

Despite these reservations, it is worth noting that such information as we have got about consumer attitudes tends to confirm the conclusion that Scotland is better able to satisfy the needs of its population. A survey conducted for the Commission on the Constitution in 1973 showed a higher proportion of respondents in Scotland (62%) saying that the hospital service in their region was 'very good' than in any other part of the United Kingdom.[26] It may also prove possible to obtain a breakdown of opinion by country of the data collected by the Royal Commission on the NHS.[27] Although it is always unsatisfactory to use data collected for one purpose for a different one, such a re-analysis of the available information may at least provide a starting point for comparative research.

A tentative conclusion

As argued at the beginning of this paper, it is crucial to be clear what the objective of any exercise in comparative research is supposed to be. In the case of social policy in England, Scotland and Northern Ireland, it is tempting to assume that the focus of analytical interest can be the relatively small variations in the structure and organisation of the social services – since environmental factors can be assumed to be relatively unimportant. The exercise then is primarily in the learning mode: the object is to test models. However, the discussion of the social, political and population factors may suggest that it is possible to reverse this argument: that the objective of the analysis might be to ask whether relatively homogeneous social services have a different effect in different environmental settings. The exercise then is primarily in the explanatory mode with the emphasis on political and social rather than organisational variables. Whichever approach is adopted, it has been argued that the research strategy should be to concentrate on specific issues, rather than to attempt to make a general comparison of organisations and structure. But a further conclusion might also be that a research strategy for comparative research should look beyond England, Scotland and Northern Ireland – since only by enlarging the sample of countries for study will it be possible to come to any conclusions about such environmental variables as size and basic, as distinct from marginal, differences in the organisational structure, financial basis and ideological bias of the social services.

Notes

1. This section draws heavily on: T. R. Marmor, A. Bridges and W. L. Hoffman 'Comparative politics and health policies', paper presented for conference at Cornell University, 14 October 1976, mimeo.
2. See for example H. N. Bunbury (ed.), *Lloyd George's Ambulance Wagon: the Memoirs of William J. Braithwaite*, Bath: Cedric Chivers Ltd., 1957.
3. Committee on One-Parent Families, *Report and Appendices*, London: HMSO, 1974.

4. H. L. Wilensky, *The Welfare State and Equality*, Berkeley: University of California Press, 1975; P. Flora, J. Alber and J. Kohl, 'Zur Entwicklung der West-Europaischen Wohlfahrstsstaaten', *Politische Vierteljahressschrift*, Vol. 18, no. 4, 1977; J. Carrier and I. Kendall, 'The Development of Welfare States: the production of plausible accounts', *Journal of Social Policy*, Vol. 6 Part 3, July, 1977.
5. H. Eckstein, *Pressure Group Politics*, London: Allen and Unwin, 1960.
6. T. R. Marmor and D. Thomas, 'Doctors, Politics and Pay Disputes', *British Journal of Political Science*, October 1972.
7. Outstandingly, H. Heclo, *Modern Social Politics in Britain and Sweden*, New Haven, Conn.: Yale University Press, 1974.
8. The phrase is taken from D. Braybrooke, *Traffic Congestion goes through the issue-machine*, London: Routledge and Kegan Paul, 1974.
9. M. Rein, *Social Science and Public Policy*, Harmondsworth, Penguin, 1976.
10. Wilensky, 1975.
11. For example, J. Higgins, *The Poverty Business*, Oxford: Basil Blackwell/Martin Robertson, 1978.
12. R. Rose, *Governing without consensus*, London: Faber, 1971.
13. M. Buxton and R. Klein, *Allocating health resources*, Royal Commission on the NHS Research Paper No. 3, London: HMSO, 1978.
14. For a general review, see OECD *Public Expenditure on Health*, Paris: OECD, July 1977.
15. A. J. Kahn and S. B. Kamerman, *Social Services in International Perspective*, Washington DC: US Department of Health, Education and Welfare, 1976.
16. J. Blanpain *et al.*, *National Health Insurance and Health Resources*, Cambridge, Mass: Harvard University Press, 1978; A. Maynard, *Health Care in the European Community*, London: Croom Helm, 1975; I. Douglas Wilson and G. McLachlan (eds.), *Health Service Prospects*, Nuffield Provincial Hospitals Trust, 1973.
17. R. Kohn and K. L. White, *Health Care: Report of the World Health Organisation International Collaborative Study of Medical Care Utilisation*, Oxford: Oxford University Press, 1976.
18. O. W. Anderson, *Health Care: can there be equity*, New York: John Wiley, 1972.
19. T. R. Marmor, D. A. Wittman and T. C. Heagy, 'Politics, Public Policy and Medical Inflation', in M. Zubkoff (ed.), *Health: A Victim or Cause of Inflation?*, Milbank Memorial Fund, 1976.
20. A. P. Zhuk, *Public Health Planning in the USSR*, Washington, DC: US Department of Health, Education and Welfare, 1976.
21. M. Kogan *et al.*, *The working of the National Health Service*, Royal Commission on the NHS Working Paper no. 1, London: HMSO, 1978.
22. L. A. Aday, 'Economic and noneconomic barriers to the use of needed medical services', *Medical Care*, Vol. 13, no. 6, June 1975.
23. Here the model would be studies such as A. I. Harris, *Social Welfare for the Elderly*, London: HMSO 1968.
24. For example, M. Blaxter, 'Social class and health inequalities', in C. O. Carter and J. Peel (eds.), *Equalities and Inequalities in Health*, London: Academic Press, 1976.
25. See, however, Elizabeth Collins and Rudolf Klein, 'Equity and the NHS: self-reported morbidity, access and primary care', *British Medical Journal*, 25 October 1980.
26. Commission on the Constitution Research Papers no. 7, *Devolution and other aspects of Government: an Attitudes Survey*, London: HMSO, 1973.
27. J. Gregory, *Patients' attitudes to the Hospital Service*, Royal Commission on the NHS Research Paper no. 5, London: HMSO, 1978.

3 Comparative Social Policy Research and the Components of the United Kingdom

Fred Martin

Whether or not there is a case for planning comparative social policy research between the component parts of the United Kingdom must depend on our objectives in embarking on comparative studies at all.

Comparative observations and analysis can be carried out with brushstrokes of varying thickness. At one extreme we can take a global view and with truly Olympian detachment differentiate between very broad categories of social, economic and administrative systems. From this standpoint we can, for example, speak of welfare capitalism and lump together a dozen or more societies, contrasting them perhaps to the centrally planned economies. Given such a broad distinction the differences between, say, Britain and Denmark and West Germany become trivial, while the differences between England and Scotland pale into insignificance. The fine detail, from this perspective, becomes irrelevant, and the scrutiny of it a waste of time which could be more productively spent in ideologically-related generalisation.

Most comparative research however is conceived and carried out within a narrower international framework, often limiting itself to Western capitalist and mixed economies, and examining ways in which different countries have gone about solving what are seen as more or less common problems. Much of this work is essentially descriptive. We tend to say of the fruits of these labours that they are 'useful', but we're not always quite sure just what it is they are useful *for*. Their most obvious value is that they provide a check on ethnocentrism, reminding us that familiar ways of responding to a given set of needs or problems – or even familiar ways of conceptualising needs and problems – are not the only possible ways. Yet with the best will in the world, our ability to profit from such studies, in the sense of drawing lessons which are potentially applicable on the domestic scene, is often severely restricted.

Barbara Rodgers comments:

> One would expect that many of those who write for pressure groups, or who are in some other way politically committed to some general or specific scheme for advancing the welfare of a particular citizen group in their country, might be something less than objective in their analysis of the political,

> economic and administrative implications of the measures they advocate. But when they look at apparently comparable measures and achievements of another country, the political, economic and administrative concomitants for that country and its almost certainly different economic, social, cultural, demographic and political history and geography are more often than not left right out of the account.[1]

But when the multiplicity of concomitant factors *is* taken into account, we may well conclude that the particular policy or practice in which we are ultimately interested is so interwoven with other and distinctive aspects of that society and its culture that its chances of surviving transplantation into an alternative environment are quite slender.

Most, though not all, such comparative studies are overly dependent on what might be termed administrative descriptions of service provision, leavened to some extent by the commentaries derived from critical literature. One obvious difficulty in this context is that comparative studies that do not generate their own data are inevitably dependent on the quantity and quality of research and analysis carried out by others; and these may well have considerable limitations, resulting either from mere lack of research interest or from political inhibition. For example, anyone who was interested in the social security system of the United Kingdom could be referred not only to the legislation and the formal descriptive material provided by the official agencies, but also to shelves of research reports and critical analyses by workers who have questioned bland official assumptions, and set out to identify the gaps, the failures and the weaknesses of the system. It does seem to be very much more difficult to gain access to comparative critical data relating to, say, the countries of Eastern Europe. To take a specific example, anyone who is interested in the continuing role of the private sector in medical care within a predominantly state-based system can without excessive difficulty assemble a reasonably clear descriptive account of the position in this country. How feasible a task would this be in Poland, for example? As far as I can gather, the official literature does not recognise that private medical care even exists, though my personal impression is that it operates on a very substantial scale. (I vividly recall a conversation in Warsaw about fifteen years ago with a distinguished Polish sociologist, who made the point that in a one-party system there was a special responsibility on the social sciences to take on some of the functions of an opposition, and submit official policies to critical ssrutiny; and that this was possible within certain limits because the ethos of science still carried weight. But that particular period of liberal tolerance came to an end quite soon afterwards.)

When we come to consider the component parts of the United Kingdom we have to paint with very fine brush-strokes indeed. Most of the obvious differences between social, economic and political systems which complicate international comparisons have been, in the statistician's phrase, partialled out. The fact that there are differences between the component parts in respect of, say, the incidence of poverty, the characteristic patterns of housing tenure and the overall levels of mortality and morbidity, though relevant and not to be ignored is not really crucial. These I think are regional considerations and would need equally to be taken into account if one were looking at Lancashire in comparison with Sussex. The points of departure for comparative studies are differences in legislation, in administrative structure of services, in planned and unplanned interrelations between areas of service provision. The application of these criteria would suggest that Wales was not appropriately differentiated from England and should not therefore be considered a separate element for purposes of comparative social policy research.

In his contribution to this volume, Professor Klein takes the view that the differences may be too small to make comparative study profitable anywhere within the UK. This is probably quite a widely shared view, and is in harmony with the practice of all existing English textbooks on social services or social administration to deal exclusively with the situation in England and Wales, dismissing the eccentricities of Scotland – and sometimes Northern Ireland – in a slightly irritated footnote. It is not an opinion which I can go along with, although I would agree that the scope for such studies is comparatively limited, limited that is to work at the micro level. This may be no bad thing. We may have an opportunity here to get away from the 'so what?' that greets much comparative descriptive research. When so many factors are held constant, it may become a little easier to consider not what policies *are*, but what they *do*. To say this, however, is to be reminded how painfully limited are the measures we have at present for understanding policy outputs, their quality, their impact and their effectiveness. I'm not sure that academics have been very much less reticent than politicians in displaying the Oliver Twist syndrome. We tend to have our own areas of special concern, our own favoured client groups, and to argue for more inputs – more money, more personnel, bigger services. We have little by which to judge the benefits derived from varying levels or types of input. Occasionally we can pick up a revealing if ambiguous disparity in basic statistics and ask pertinent questions – for example, when we look at the relatively high level of expenditure on health services in Scotland, or the relatively favourable doctor-patient ratio, and contrast these with the comparatively unfavourable mortality and morbidity statistics. We may of course see that high level of expenditure as an appropriate response to a high level of need. More plausibly, however, we might question whether the ways in which health services are patterned and delivered are as well attuned to the prevailing health care needs and their social context as they might be. Yet again, we might take the view that the underlying causes of illness and premature death in Scotland are so deeply rooted in social conditions that concentration on health services expenditure diverts resources from alternative applications which might conceivably prove more effective. My aim is not to pre-judge this particular issue, merely to point out that this is one of the comparatively few instances in which we have a measure of outcome, albeit of the simplest and most basic kind. For the most part, we need to develop sensitive and specialised measures for assessing the quality of services and the consequences of their delivery. This is scarcely an unfamiliar plea. It arises whenever one looks at the problem of controlled evaluation studies, though it is by no means the only problem that needs to be solved in that area. But if we cannot make significant progress on that front, I do not see very much scope for comparative social policy research as between the components of the United Kingdom.

At the best, the issues we can hope to tackle will be fairly modest ones, related to variations arising from differences in legislation, in administrative structure, in policy initiatives within a common legislative structure or in what can only be called long-term preferences or orientations which may never have been formulated as explicit policies. A few examples of researchable questions falling under these headings may serve to illustrate their range.

One important element in the implementation of the Social Work (Scotland) Act was an agreement by the Scottish probation service to accept euthanasia. When however the Seebohm Committee was established at about the same time to review the future of personal social services in England and Wales, the probation service was explicitly excluded from its terms of reference. As a result, therefore, we continue to have a substantial and separate probation service south of the border, while probation officers in Scotland, with the exception of those who took up new posts such as reporters to children's panels, were absorbed into local authority social work departments as generic social workers. Indeed, as the largest group of trained workers to be incorporated into the new service, former probation officers took up a significant proportion of the management positions created by the reorganisation of personal social services. Here we have two quite clear and opposite policy decisions, based on different assumptions about social work and about the management of offenders. And it is pertinent to ask whether they have made any perceptible difference to anyone.

I think the impact on the professionals concerned is by no means the most momentous aspect, though it would be of some interest to examine the subsequent careers and present job satisfaction of two ten-year-old cohorts of probation officers. But a good deal more important in reviewing the outcome of decisions made a decade ago would be a study which began with a series of offenders who had been put under the care of probation officers in England, and attempted to match this with a series of offenders in Scotland comparable in terms of say age, type of offence and previous offence history. How was this second group dealt with? Can we compare the content and meaning of any supervisory relationship in the two very different work situations? Such comparisons would be fraught with methodological difficulties but would be well worth attempting, though to go on to ask questions about outcomes might involve unmanageable burdens. If we cannot tease out some identifiable patterns of variation associated with and flowing from contrasting policy decisions, we shall need to examine extremely sceptically the judgements on which those decisions were based.

Studies of policy innovations can scarcely ever be mounted on a truly experimental basis. It is important therefore to seek out naturally occurring experiments or quasi-experiments which give us the nearest approximation to experimental situations that we can normally hope to find. While one could never suggest that in a comparison of specific English and Scottish developments it is possible to assume that all other factors were constant, one is certainly able to hold at bay those massive variations in history, in social structure and culture which invalidate so many cross-national comparisons of social policy.

The second example is in a field that is not generally thought of as a social service, though it is certainly a proper concern of social policy. In England and Wales the overwhelming majority of criminal prosecutions are initiated by the police, with the Director of Public Prosecutions being involved only in cases which are serious or of particular public importance. Scottish practice on the other hand is quite different; the office of procurator-fiscal is of long standing, and he acts in effect as a public prosecutor in the ordinary sheriff courts. Nor does the procurator-fiscal prosecute automatically, on receipt of instructions from the police. The police refer cases to him, and he uses his own criteria to decide whether a prosecution should or should not be instituted. The procurator-fiscal service is a substantial one, employing some forty full-time lawyers in the city of Glasgow alone. In recent years the practice of the police acting as a prosecuting as well as a law enforcement agency has come under very considerable criticism, and has been considered by the Royal Commission on Criminal Procedure (1978–81, Cmnd no. 8092). There is on the face of it a striking Anglo-Scottish difference. How significant a difference is it? How does the procurator-fiscal function, particularly in his discretionary role, and in what concrete ways are the administration of justice and its consequences affected by the existence of this distinctive agency? The way in which the Scottish system operates has never, as far as I know, been studied in any systematic fashion.[2] Possibly it is jealously guarded against the prying curiosity of researchers. But it seems to me there is scope for genuinely comparative study in an area where quite different procedures have evolved out of complex historical tradition and not as a result of any explicit policy decisions. Whether the different patterns have developed separately to such an extent that some equivalent of the Scottish prosecuting system would be quite unacceptable within an English context is arguable. But even if that seemed the likely outcome, it would still be of great interest to examine the relations between police and fiscals, the ways in which comparable types of case are processed in the two systems, the criteria applied and the broader legal and social consequences.

It seems likely that the office of procurator-fiscal provided a model for the local goverment official known as the reporter to the children's panel, who plays a key role in the juvenile justice system establshed in Scotland under Part III of the Social Work (Scotland) Act. Structurally at any rate the Scottish system is entirely different from that which prevails elsewhere in the UK, and it represents one of the few instances in which there has been a quite major deviation in social policy as between London and Edinburgh. The formal differences do not need to be discussed here in any detail, but it is relevant to ask what these differences affect and what is actually experienced by the child and his parents. Does the Scottish system, with its built-in provisions for diversion, its lay volunteer component, its explicit commitment to an ideology of care (though not exclusively of 'treatment'), in fact produce less stigma, less labelling, less recidivism? It would be of fascinating interest to know. Some fairly intensive studies of Scottish hearings system have recently been carried out involving analyses of the discretionary decision-making activities of both reporters and panel members, the use made of professional reports, the processes of interaction that go on in the hearing itself, the subjective reactions of clients, and the attitudinal patterns of panel members,[3] but research that is planned to be even broadly comparative seems still to be a long way off.

During the 1960s English psychiatric hospitals embarked on – or perhaps it would be more accurate to say were committed to – a policy of 'run-down'. It was intended by the central department that the number of beds in psychiatric hospitals and units should be reduced by one-half during the next dozen years, with a strong emphasis on decanting as many as possible of the existing long-stay population as rapidly as possible, and on establishing short-term treatment and early discharge as the norm for new admissions. In the event the process of 'running-down' proved to be a good deal slower than had been planned, but even so there is no doubt that by now a very substantial shift has been achieved. In Scotland the trend has been considerably and deliberately slower, in spite of the fact that the initial level of in-patient provision was significantly higher than in England. This striking variation in pace was not attributable to legislative differences, but to administrative and professional decisions of a more cautious and conservative kind. Is it possible to make any statement about the ways in which the clinical and social histories of the mentally ill north and south of the border have been affected by quite marked differences in the ways in which hospital provision has been used? To the best of my knowledge, it has never even been suggested that some research attention might be justified. But it should not be insuperably difficult to begin by comparing the distributions of diagnoses among admissions, discharges and out-patients at different times; and then to examine within diagnostic groups variations in hospital career, in experience in the community, in burdens on families. Both English and Scottish policies arose from beliefs about the advantages of doing things this way rather than that way, but no one has thought it worthwhile to attempt to estimate the comparative validity of those beliefs.

All examples so far suggested have been Anglo-Scottish, reflecting the writer's personal interests. But Northern Ireland sometimes offers striking variations, and in spite of its small scale and internal conflicts it should not be excluded from any programme of comparative studies. To take a single but very important example: health services and social services seem on the face of it to have a degree of formal integration which has no parallel in Great Britain. Many commentators however have remarked on the adverse effects of the segregation of social from health services, and have drawn attention to the discontinuities that this may create for a number of client groups. Some medical critics have argued for the complete integration of the two services, though in general their views have been rejected by spokesmen for the social work profession and social service organisations, partly because of a belief that integration is a polite euphemism for medical domination. Even when complete unification is not advocated, however, there is strong encouragement to cooperate and coordinate. While the prevailing pattern of services in Northern Ireland would need to be examined in its own right, (see Chapter 8 of this volume), a comparative element would be of great value. Again I would argue that a major emphasis should be on outcomes and consequences, and not merely on intentions and assumptions. The way in which different services actually operate and the results that their ways of working have for specified client groups would require examination in the context of both Northern Ireland and England or Scotland. Child health, the care of the elderly, services for the mentally ill, the mentally handicapped and the physically disabled have all been identified at various times as areas in which divided responsibility has militated against comprehensive and continuous care. Controlled comparisons of service relationships, service delivery and consequences for clients could give some measure of the advantages and drawbacks of different organisational patterns.

Studies of the kind outlined above, though described as modest, are quite difficult to plan, to execute and to interpret. Many of the problems are conceptual and methodological, involving formulation of criteria and devices for assessing them. But even when we have worked out tentative approaches to those problems of design and interpretation about which we can learn a little from the textbooks on research methodology, we have still to come to terms with the fact that there are sometimes obstacles of quite a different order which may block the way to this particular field of study. Political and administrative sensitivities are very easily aroused. It will be assumed by those from whom rights of access must be sought that comparisons must be invidious, if not odious. A personal anecdote may illustrate this problem-area, which though not in the ordinary sense of any academic significance is nevertheless among the realities that have to be taken into account. In 1977, when we were beginning work on the study of the children's hearings system mentioned earlier, we picked up a suggestion in an official report on a serious case of non-accidental injury in the West of England, that Scottish procedures might well provide a more effective means of handling such cases. Although that statement seemed over-optimistic, I took advantage of the report to put it to the DHSS that there might be some merit in a careful comparison of the strengths and weaknesses of the different ways in which cases of suspected non-accidental injury were 'processed' on both sides of the border. I was invited to a meeting in London at which administrative, social work and research staff were all represented, the latter being drawn from the Home Office as well as the DHSS. It was a polite and amiable enough meeting, but it soon became clear that there was no possibility of DHSS support for anything resembling a comparative study. And although no one said so in as many words, I found it impossible to escape the conclusion that there was deep reluctance to embark on any investigation which might conceivably be interpreted as implying that there was anything useful to be learned from the barbarians in the North. The underlying attitudes might prove to be the most serious stumbling-block of all; and it may be worthwhile to give some thought to possible strategies for encouraging that official approval (or at least tolerance) without which comparative studies of social policy will be seriously handicapped.

Notes

1. The situation has changed since the time of writing. See S. R. Moody and J. Tombs, *Prosecution in the Public Interest*, Edinburgh: Scottish Academic Press, 1982.
2. B. Rodgers, 'Comparative studies in social policy and administration', in H. Heisler (ed.), *Foundations of Social Administration*, London: Macmillan, 1977.
3. See F. M. Martin, S. J. Fox and K. Murray, *Children out of Court*, Edinburgh: Scottish Academic Press, 1981.

PART TWO
Health and Personal Social Services

4 Health and Personal Social Services in the United Kingdom: the statutory position

Chris Himsworth

Introduction

The main purpose of this paper is to provide a statutory backdrop for discussion of the present provision of health and personal social services within the four regions (a term in this context not used disparagingly) of the UK – England, Wales, Scotland and Northern Ireland. What the paper amounts to, therefore, is substantially a comparative analysis of the principal relevant legislation (in all cases, as subsequently amended):

Social Work (Scotland) Act 1968 (the '1968 Act');
Local Authority Social Services Act 1970 (the '1970 Act');
Health and Personal Social Services (Northern Ireland) Order 1972 (SI no. 1265) (the '1972 Order');
National Health Service Act 1977 (the '1977 Act'), and the
National Health Service (Scotland) Act 1978 (the '1978) Act').
(The 1977 Act and the 1978 Act have been substantially amended by the Health Services Act 1980. This is referred to as the '1980 Act'.)

This discussion has, of course, to be supplemented by reference to subordinate legislation and to other legislation relevant to the two fields. Where it might be helpful some reference is also made to earlier legislation and, at appropriate points, the law relevant to other social services (education and housing in particular) is mentioned in order to provide a rather fuller picture.

The approach in writing the paper has been to provide a dispassionate and, even more importantly, an almost purely legal picture of the structure of the services with very little reference to the administrative structures which have been superimposed. This distinction between what is statutorily provided and what is administratively grafted on is not, however, easy to maintain and, at some points in the paper, the dividing line is crossed. Another difficulty encountered was that of maintaining some sort of coherence in the discussion of the different structures in two different services in four jurisdictions without lapsing into a chaotic intermingling of legislation or alternatively 'compartmentalising' to such an extent that comparisons cannot be made. The mode of exposition adopted has, in the event, been to divide the discussion into some seven different functional parts and then, in each part, to look at both health and personal social services in each region. The seven divisions chosen are as follows:

1. The central government authority (normally simply the minister and department responsible) and that authority's statutory functions in relation to the service.
2. Any other 'central' bodies – advisory, consultative, etc. – and their composition and functions.
3. The authorities for the local administration of the services, their composition and powers.
4. Local advisory and consultative bodies.
5. The rules governing the relationships between the bodies discussed in (1) and (3) (to the extent that they have not been already treated).
6. Institutions designed to encourage public participation in the services.
7. The extent of provision for liaison between authorities at all levels in the health, personal social services and other services.

The central government

Both the services are operated through a combination of both 'central' and 'local' administrations and the identification of the cental authority in each case is relatively straightforward. For England, the Secretary of State referred to in both the 1970 Act (Social Services) and the 1977 Act (Health) is the Secretary of State for Health and Social Services acting (with four junior ministers) through the Department of Health and Social Security. In the same Acts in relation to Wales, the relevant Secretary of State is the Secretary of State for Wales – a post created in that name as recently as 1964 and to whom responsibility for health services in Wales was delegated in 1969 (SI 1969/388) and for social services (including childcare) in 1971. The Secretary of State discharges his functions (with two junior ministers) through the Health and Social Work Department of the Welsh Office. His other functions include responsibility for primary and secondary education, housing and town and country planning in Wales.

In Scotland, the minister for the purposes of the 1968 and 1978 Acts is the Secretary of State for Scotland. He discharges his functions through the Scottish Office (with a total of four junior ministers) – in the case of health, the Scottish Home and Health Department and, in the case of social work, the Social Work Services Group of the Scottish Education Department.

In Northern Ireland, central responsibility is vested in the Department (prior to January 1974, 'Ministry' – see Northern Ireland Constitution Act 1973, s. 7) of Health and Social Services for the functions in the 1972 Order. The 1972 Order was made under the Northern Ireland (Temporary Provisions) Act 1972 in the first period of direct rule following the end of the 'Stormont system' of devolved government. Orders made under that Act, and latterly under the Northern Ireland Act 1974, now make up Northern Ireland's 'primary' legislation in most fields. The 1974 Act (s.I.(3) and Schedule 1, para 2) provides that functions of all Northern Ireland Departments be discharged subject to the direction and control of the Secretary of State (for Northern Ireland). The 1972 Order covers the provision of most health and personal social services but not, as in England and Wales, the probation and aftercare service which under the Probation Act (Northern Ireland) 1950 remains with the department responsible for law and order in the province which, under direct rule, is the Northern Ireland Office. For education and housing in Northern Ireland, the central departments are the Education and Environment Departments respectively (both subject to the political control of the Secretary of State who has four junior ministers altogether).

In both services, the central authority, whether Secretary of State or Department, has an overall responsibility for their provision although the terms of that responsibility differ – especially as between the social services in England, Wales and Scotland and the rest (health and both services in Northern Ireland). In all cases, there is a general and then a number of specific responsibilities.

For Northern Ireland the duty of the Ministry is stated to be (Art. 4):

> (a) to provide or secure the provision of integrated health services in Northern Ireland designed to promote the physical and mental health of the people of Northern Ireland through the prevention, diagnosis and treatment of illness;
> (b) to provide or secure the provision of personal social services in Northern Ireland designed to promote the social welfare of the people of Northern Ireland;
>
> and the Ministry shall so discharge its duty as to secure the effective coordination of health and personal social services.

Subsequent articles require the provision by the Ministry of *inter alia* accommodation and medical services (Art. 5); general health services (Art. 6 and Part VI); arrangements to prevent illness etc. (Art. 7); family planning services (Art. 12); educational and research facilities (Art. 13); health education (Art. 14) and general social welfare (Art. 15). In practice, of course, this provision is made by the Health and Social Services Boards which, under Art. 16, the Ministry is bound to establish (see below).

The general duties to provide a health service in England and Wales (1977 Act, s.1(1)) and Scotland 1978 Act, s.1(1)) are cast in very similar terms. Both the Acts are consolidation Acts and, therefore, in re-enacting the duties in the 1946 and 1947 Acts refer to a duty to 'continue' to provide a health service. The Scottish formulation is:

> It shall continue to be the duty of the Secretary of State to promote in Scotland a comprehensive and integrated health service designed to secure
> (a) improvement in the physical and mental health of the people of Scotland, and
> (b) the prevention, diagnosis and treatment of illness,
> and for that purpose to provide or secure the effective provision of services in accordance with the provisions of this Act.

The 1977 Act differs only slightly in making no reference to an 'integrated' service and in referring only to a duty to 'secure improvement' in the prevention etc. of illness rather than actually to secure the prevention etc.

Thereafter, the styles of the two Acts differ in that the Scottish Act moves straight on to the Secretary of State's duty to establish health boards (s.2) and other agencies before returning to his duty 'to secure the provision of general medical, general dental and general opthalmic services, and of pharmaceutical services' (s.18); to provide hospital accomodation and other services and facilities (ss. 36–48); to control prices of medical supplies (s.49) and to control the use of NHS facilities by private patients (ss. 50–64). In the 1977 Act for England and Wales, the more general functions of the Secretary of State are set out at the start (ss. 2–5) before their more detailed treatment in Parts II and III of the Act.

Because they vest primary responsibility for the provision of services in local authorities, the Acts of 1968 and 1970 make totally different provision for the Secretary of State's function. He is given a number of specific powers of supervision and control (discussed below) but no general responsibility to secure the provision of services. The nearest to such a general role is set out in the 1968 Act, s.5(1).

> Local authorities shall perform their functions under this Act under the general guidance of the Secretary of State

and in the 1970 Act, s.7(1)

> Local authorities shall, in the exercise of their social services, functions, including the exercise of any discretion conferred by any relevant enactment, act under the general guidance of the Secretary of State.

Other central bodies

This heading covers a wide range of bodies differing greatly in composition. Perhaps the most useful distinction is that between executive and purely advisory or consultative bodies. To clarify subsequent discussion the more important ones will first be listed under those two heads

Executive

1. Medical Practices Committee (Health, England and Wales) (1977 Act, s.7)
2. Scottish Medical Practices Committee (Health, Scotland) (1978 Act, s.3)
3. Dental Estimates Board (Health, England and Wales) (1977 Act, s.37)
4. Scottish Dental Estimates Board (Health, Scotland) (1978 Act, s.4)
5. Common Services Agency (Health, Scotland) (1978 Act, s.10 and Sched. 5).
6. Northern Ireland Central Services Agency for the Health and Social Services (1972 Order, Art. 26)
7. Welsh Health Technical Services Organisation and its Welsh Pricing Committee (1977 Act, s.11 and SI 1973/1624)
8. Prescription Pricing Authority (Health, England) (1977 Act, s.11 and SI 1974/9)
9. Public Health Laboratory Service Board (Health, England and Wales) (1977 Act, s.5 and Sched. 3 as amended by the Public Health Laboratory Service Act 1979)
10. Scottish Hospital Trust (1978 Act, s.11)
12. The Tribunal (disqualifications) (Health, England and Wales) (1977 Act, s.46)
13. The Tribunal (Scottish) (1978 Act, s.29)
14. The United Kingdom Central Council for Nursing, Midwifery and Health Visiting (Nurses, Midwives and Health Visitors Act 1979 which dissolved the Central Midwives Boards for England and Wales and Scotland, the two General Nursing Councils, the Northern Ireland Council for Nurses and Midwives and the Council for the Education and Training of Health Visitors). There are also National Boards for Nursing, Midwifery and Health Visiting for each of the four regions.
15. General Dental Council (UK)
16. General Medical Council (UK) (Medical Act 1956)
17. General Optical Council (UK) (Opticians Act 1958)
18. General Practice Finance Corporation (England, Wales and Scotland) (National Health Service Act 1966 as amended by the 1980 Act)
19. Council for Education and Training in Social Work (UK) (Health Visiting and Social Work (Training) Act 1962) and its Scotland and Northern Ireland Advisory Committees.

The Health Services Board established by the Health Services Act 1976, s.1 was abolished by the 1980 Act, s.9.

Advisory/consultative

1. Standing Medical, Nursing and Midwifery, Dental, Pharmaceutical and Opthalmic Advisory Committees (Health, England and Wales) (1977 Act, s.6) (The Central Health Services Council was dissolved by the 1980 Act, s.8)
2. Scottish Health Service Planning Council (1978 Act, s.5 and Sched. 3) and national (professional) consultative committees (s.6)
3. Northern Ireland Health and Social Services Council (1972 Order, Art. 22)

Note: The Advisory Council on Social Work (Scotland) was abolished by the Local Government (Miscellaneous Provisions) (Scotland) Act 1981, s.29. There was also from 1973 a non-statutory Personal Social Services Council for England and Wales, but that too has been dissolved.

It would be impossible in a paper of this kind to contemplate discussion of the composition and functions of all these bodies. A selective approach has to be taken. On the 'executive' side the most important are probably the common services agencies. A note on these, and then on the advisory bodies, follows.

The common services agencies Here we are talking about the Scottish Common Services Agency, the Welsh Health Technical Services Organisation and the Northern Ireland Central Services Agency for the Health and Social Services.

The Scottish Agency is now established (although originally under the NHS (Scotland) Act 1972) in terms of s.10 and Schedule 5 of the 1978 Act supplemented by rules as to membership and procedure in SI 1975/196 and as to functions in SI 1974/467. The Agency is constituted as a body corporate to be managed by a management committee consisting of a chairman appointed by the Secretary of State, five further members appointed by the Secretary of State, a further six similarly appointed but on the nomination of the Health Boards acting jointly, and such other members as the Secretary of State may appoint after consultation with the Health Boards. Rules as to terms of office, resignations, and procedure (including disabilities from voting) are set out in SI 1975/196. The Agency is empowered to employ staff.

The functions of the Agency are those determined by the Secretary of State. He may delegate some of his own functions and he may, after consultation with the Planning Council and Health Boards, order that Health Board functions may stand referred to the Agency to be discharged by it on behalf of any or all of the Boards in the interests of efficiency. Regulations (SI 1974/467) now require of the Agency *inter alia* the general provision of accommodation and services as required by the Secretary of State or by Health Boards, the procurement of equipment and supplies, the provision of information and health education, the provision of an ambulance service, the coordination of personnel policies and staff training, and the provision of legal services to Health Boards.

The Welsh Health Technical Services Organisation discharges many of the same functions for Wales. Under s.11 of the 1977 Act the Secretary of State is empowered to establish special health authorities to perform functions on his own behalf or on behalf of an Area Health Authority or Family Practitioner Committee. This power has been exercised (SI 1974/9 as amended) to establish for England the Prescription Pricing Authority to carry out the functions of checking and pricing prescriptions on behalf of Family Practitioner Committees. The membership is drawn from four prescribed groups of the Committees. For Wales, however, the same power was used to establish (SI 1973/1624) the wider ranging Technical Services Organisation. It is composed of a chairman and between six and eight other members appointed by the Secretary of State. Of these three must be appointed on the nomination of the Area Health Authorities (acting together) and up to two may be appointed after consultation with the authorities. Functions are what the Secretary of State directs within a range prescribed in the order including functions relating to capital works, the procurement of supplies, the provision of computer services and the checking and pricing of supplies, the provision of computer services and the checking and pricing of prescriptions. For this last purpose, the Order requires the appointment of the Organisation, two members representative of registered pharmacists, one member representative of medical practitioners, and two members nominated by Family Practitioner Committees.

Statutory provision for the Northern Ireland Central Services Agency for Health and Social Services is more skeletal. Its establishment is required by the 1972 Order, Art. 26 and Schedule 3, and it is composed of a chairman and vice-chairman both to be appointed by the Minister (now Secretary of State) and such other members as he may appoint following consultation with the Health and Social Services Boards and other interests. The Agency's functions are such of the Department's own functions as the Department directs and such of the Board's functions as, after consultation with them, the Department considers expedient for efficiency.

Advisory bodies Remaining in Northern Ireland, the relevant advisory bodies are the Health and Social Services Council (Arts. 22–23 and Schedule 2) and the central and other advisory committees (Arts. 24–25). The membership of the Council is a chairman and vice-chairman appointed by the Secretary of State, the chairman and one other member of each Board, the chairman of each central advisory committee, and others appointed after consultation with universities and other interests. Its functions are to advise the two relevant departments on the exercise of their functions; to keep under review the development and coordination of health and personal social services generally and, if directed by the Department, to make an annual report. Central advisory committees for professions engaged in relevant services may be appointed by the Secretary of State for the purpose of advising the Council and also to carry out investigations on behalf of the Council.

In Great Britain, provision for advisory councils and committees divides between services and regions. So far as health is concerned, England and Wales on the one hand and Scotland on the other have the standing advisory committees (and until the 1980 Act, the Central Health Services Council) and the Scottish Health Service Planning Council and national consultative committees respectively.

The standing advisory committees are appointed by the Secretary of State under s.6(3) (as amended by the 1980 Act, s.8[2]) (the NHS [Standing Advisory Committee] Order as amended by SI 1974/196). They are listed above and have the duty to advise the Secretary of State on the services with which they are concerned.

The Scottish Health Service Planning Council (1978 Act, s.5 and Sched. 3) has functions similar to those of the Central Council. It has, however, a different composition with a chairman appointed by the Secretary of State, a member appointed by each of the fifteen Health Boards, a member appointed by each University with a medical school, and up to six members appointed by the Secretary of State. The Scottish National Consultative Committees (1978 Act, s.6) have similar statutory functions to their English counterparts although the 'renumeration and conditions of service of practitioners' are specifically excluded from their remit. Powers to specify further the Committees' functions have not been exercised. The Committees are brought into existence not by order but simply through their 'recognition' by the Secretary of State as committees representative of professions.

In the personal social services, there has been considerable change in the last few years as a result of 'quango culling'. The former Advisory Council on Social Work (Scotland) and the Personal Social Services Council (England and Wales) have disappeared. There remains, however, for England and Wales the Advisory Council on Child Care (Child Care

Act 1980, s.71) appointed by the Secretary of State and advising him in connection with his child care functions.

Local administrative authorities

This section provides a sketch of the authorities concerned with the local administration of services. These are, for England, Wales and Scotland, the social services and social work authorities for the purposes of the 1970 and 1968 Acts and the health authorities and boards under the Acts of 1977 and 1978. For Northern Ireland, the functions are united in the boards established by the 1972 Order.

Social Services (England and Wales)

For the purposes of the 1970 Act, social services authorities are the non-metropolitan counties, the metropolitan districts, the London boroughs and the Common Council of the City of London (1970 Act, s.1 as amended by the Local Government Act 1972, s.195). The authorities are required (1970 Act s.2 as amended by the Local Government, Planning and Land Act 1980, s.183) to discharge their functions through a social services committee (which, along with education and police committees, is one of the very few continuing mandatory committees). Non-members of the authority may be appointed to a social services committee, although a majority of the committee must be members (1970 Act, s.5). Authorities are also obliged to appoint a director of social services (s.6 as amended by the Local Government etc. Act 1980 s.183).

The main effect of the 1970 Act was the integration within one social services authority, committee and department of the previously diverse local authority welfare and childcare functions. The social service functions are those set out in the Schedule 1 and include powers and duties under the National Assistance Act 1948, the Child Care Act 1980 and the Chronically Sick and Disabled Persons Act.

For the most part social services authorities are also education authorities (with the principal exception of the ILEA). Local housing powers are vested in district authorities and thus, outside the metropolitan areas, are separated from the social services.

Social Work (Scotland)

The 1968 Act integrated personal social service functions in Scotland which, upon local government reorganisation in 1975, were vested in the new regional and island councils (1968 Act, s.1 and Local Government (Scotland) Act 1973, s.161). They too are obliged to appoint social work committees and to appoint directors of social work (1968 Act, ss.2–3 as amended).

In contrast to the 1970 Act, the 1968 Act substantially re-enacts many of the local social work functions rather than simply enumerating earlier powers. The principal duties are the general promotion of social welfare by making available advice, guidance and assistance (including cash and accommodation) (s.12), the protection of children (including functions related to the children's panel system) (ss. 15–26 and Part III), and the provision of the probation service (s.27) – the most prominent departure from the English system. All social work authorities are also education authorities but, with the exception of the all-purpose islands councils, housing functions are hived off to the second-tier district councils.

Social Services and Health (Northern Ireland)

In Northern Ireland, local government was reorganised in 1973 (Local Government Act (Northern Ireland) 1972) but with the powers of the new district councils heavily reduced. Housing was transferred to the new Housing Executive (Housing Executive Act (Northern Ireland) 1971); education and library services went to new Boards (Education and Libraries (Northern Ireland) Order 1972, SI 1263); and social services were transferred with a reorganised health service to the Department and Boards of Health and Social Services (1972 Order). The Boards themselves are established by the Department for such areas as it determines. The Health and Personal Social Services (Establishment and Determination of Areas of Health and Social Services Boards) Order (Northern Ireland) 1972 (No. 217) set up the four boards and specified their areas. The constitution of the boards and the procedures they should adopt are spelled out in the 1972 Order (Arts. 16–19 and Schedule 1). Each board must consist of a chairman and vice chairman appointed by the Secretary of State; at least one person nominated by each of the district councils in the area of the Board; and further persons appointed after consultation with relevant professions, universities and other bodies. The Board must set up a Health Services Committee and a Personal Social Services Committee and may delegate functions to these and other committees. Committees may include non-members of the Board. There is further provision for the establishment of sub-committees (by Boards) and of joint committees (by the Department). The Department can require a Board to submit to the Department for its approval a scheme for the exercise of its functions.

The actual functions of the Boards are defined in the 1972 Order, Art. 17 as the general health services (i.e. general medical, dental, ophthalmic and pharmaceutical services) set out in Part VI of the Order, such services under the Adoption Act (Northern Ireland) 1967 and Children and Young Persons Act (Northern Ireland) 1968 as the NI Office directs, and such further health and social service functions as the Department directs.

Health (Scotland)

In Scotland, the equivalent health service functions are discharged by Health Boards established under the 1978 Act. Under s.2(1), the Secretary of State is required to determine Health Board areas and then, by separate order, to establish Boards for these areas. This he has done in terms of SI 1974/266 which defines the fifteen areas and SI 1974/267 which constitutes the Boards and fixes the maximum total number of members for each. There is one Board for each of the twelve Regions and Islands Areas in Scotland except the Strathclyde Region which has four Boards. The Boards are bodies corporate and consist of a chairman and members (up to the total defined in SI 1974/267) appointed by the Secretary of State. In making appointments, the Secretary of State must consult with each local authority in the Board's area, any university appearing to have an interest in health service provision in the area, representatives of medical and other professions in the area and any other organisations that appear to be concerned. The chairman of each Health Board can be paid (Schedule 1). There is further provision (s.2 and Schedule 1) for the appointment of officers by Boards; to enable the Secretary of State to issue regulations and directions according to which Boards must carry out their functions and to require Boards to submit to him schemes for the exercise of those functions. (It is in these schemes – and not in the Act itself nor in orders under it – that provision is made for the division of the areas of most Boards into districts and for the delegation of Board functions to the district administration.) The Secretary of State can, by order, establish joint committees of Boards for the purpose of carrying out some, but not all, of their functions (see SI 1974/503 which establishes three Joint Ophthalmic Committees to which the responsibilities of all Boards for the provision of general ophthalmic services are delegated).

Scottish Health Boards are required to make provision for the general medical (with no statutory equivalent of the Family Practitioner Committees in England and Wales) and other services set out in Part II of the 1978 Act. Added to these are the functions of the Secretary of State under the Act which he may by order allocate to the Boards. Such functions are prescribed in SI 1974/466 and include the provision of accommodation, premises and services (1978 Act, s.36), making arrangements for the purpose of the prevention of illness etc. (s.37), the care of mothers and young children (s.38), medical and dental inspections of children (s.39), vaccination and immunisation (s.40), family planning (s.41), health education (s.42), etc.

Health (England and Wales)

The local administration of health services in England and Wales is different and, at the time of writing, is once again in a state of flux as a result of the Health Services Act 1980. Since the terms of the 1980 Act are framed simply to permit changes to be made rather than to effect changes and since it is not yet quite certain how the powers will be used, the description which follows is of the existing system under the 1977 Act and a note on the system likely to be substantially introduced in April 1982 under the 1980 Act is appended.

The Secretary of State is required to divide England into regions and then those regions and Wales as a whole into areas and to establish for each region and area a Regional or Area Health Authority (s.8). The whole of each English area must be in a single region and the Secretary of State must ensure that each region can conveniently be associated with a university with a medical school or with two or more such universities. In contrast to Scotland and Northern Ireland, an Area Authority may be designated an Area Health Authority (Teaching) if the Secretary of State is satisfied that it is to provide for a university or universities substantial facilities for undergraduate or postgraduate clinical teaching (ss. 8–9). (The NHS Reorganisation Act 1973 abolished all the earlier health authorities although in terms of s.15 and SI 1974/281 the Boards of Governors of certain Teaching Hospitals were temporarily preserved.) Orders made under the Act establish the fourteen English Regions (SI 1973/1191), the ninety English Areas (including nineteen Teaching) and the eight Welsh Areas (including one Teaching) (SI 1973/1275). Provision is made for the establishment of the authorities and for their composition in SI 1975/1100 (Regional Authorities) and SI 1975/1099 (Area Authorities). The first order simply constitutes a Regional Authority for each region. The size of the Authorities is not defined, but all members are appointed by the Secretary of State following statutorily required consultation with local authorities, universities, professional bodies, workers' organisations and the Authority itself. This requirement to consult may be suspended by order (see SI 1977/1103).

The composition of Area Health Authorities is more closely regulated

(Schedule 5, para. 2 and SI 1975/1099). The chairman is appointed by the Secretary of State and he prescribes the total membership (18–33). Of these a specified number (1–3) are appointed by the Regional Authority on the nomination of a specified university; a further specified number (4–11) are appointed by a specified local authority (or authorities); and the remainder are appointed by the Regional Authority after consultation with professional and other bodies and the Area Authority concerned. Additional members with teaching hospital experience are appointed to Area Health Authorities (Teaching). In these rules, as they apply to Wales, the Secretary of State is the appointing body in place of the Regional Authority.

The procedure to be adopted by authorities in the discharge of their functions, including the power to delegate to committees and subcommittees is set out in the 1977 Act and SI 1973/1286. The functions themselves are prescribed partly in the 1977 Act, partly in orders made under the Act (ss. 13–18 and see especially SI 1974/24) and partly in directions authorised by the Act or orders and addressed by the Secretary of State to health authorities in general or by Regional Authorities to Area Authorities. The principal functions of Area Authorities are set out in the 1977 Act, Part II – the general medical, dental, etc. services for their areas. In terms of SI 1974/24, Regional Authorities have delegated to them practically all the Secretary of State's general health service powers (see above) so far as they relate to their region and, with certain limitations, they have the power to further delegate functions to Area Authorities by direction.

As in Scotland, administration of health services at a district level is not a formal (statutory) requirement. What is, however, required by the 1977 Act is the establishment by each Area Health Authority of a Family Practitioner Committee (s.10), an independent body corporate, whose duty is to administer on behalf of the Authority its arrangements for the provision of general health services for the area (s.15). These Committees have a normal total membership of thirty (Schedule 5, para. 6) with eleven appointed by the Area Authority (at least one, but not every one, being a member of the Authority); four by relevant local authorities; and the remainder by the local professional committees (the largest number of eight being appointed by the Local Medical Committee). Further rules on the membership, constitution and procedure of these Committees are contained in SI 1973/2012.

That, then, is the position prior to the implementation of the 1980 Act. What that Act does is to amend s.8 of the 1977 Act to provide that regions in England and Wales as a whole need no longer consist wholly of areas with Area Authorities (s.1). Instead there may be created districts with District Health Authorities or District Health Authorities (Teaching).

Thus the Secretary of State is empowered to replace Area Authorities with smaller District Authorities (having the same functions as Area Authorities). The power could be used to remove all Area Authorities or alternatively to retain some Authorities while District Authorities are created elsewhere. It is understood that, from April 1982, there will be a complete or nearly complete pattern of district Authorities.

The one other important administrative provision in the 1980 Act is that which authorises the establishment of Family Practitioner Committees for combinations of areas or districts rather than for each area as at present (s.2).

Local advisory and consultative bodies

Here we are looking primarily at the health service and at the local equivalents of the national planning and advisory bodies. For England and Wales the relevant provisions are s.19 and Schedule 6 of the 1977 Act. Under s.19 the Secretary of State is bound to 'recognise' committees both at the Regional/Welsh and Area and District levels where he is satisfied that they are representative of local medical practitioners, dental practitioners, nurses and midwives, pharmacists and opticians. Schedule 6 permits similar recognition of other professional categories. The duty of the Welsh local advisory committees is to advise the Secretary of State on the provision of services relevant to them and to perform any other prescribed functions. The other advisory committees have the same functions in relation to the Regional, Area and District Health Authorities. Virtually identical provision is made for Scotland in the 1978 Act, s.9 except, of course, that the committees exist only at the one level of the Health Board (although called *area* committees) and that consultation with Health Boards is specifically required before the recognition of committees by the Secretary of State. As at the national level, local committees in Scotland are specifically precluded from concerning themselves with remuneration and conditions of service. In addition to these local consultative committees, there should also be mentioned the Secretary of State's power under the 1978 Act, s.8 to constitute University Liaison Committees for the purpose of advising Health Boards on health service provision so far as it relates to university teaching. (There are no Health Boards specifically designated as Teaching Boards equivalent to the Area Health Authorities (Teaching) in England and Wales.) Members of these committees (Schedule 4) would be appointed in part by the Board and in part by the relevant University. In fact the power to establish these Committees has not been exercised although, on an unofficial basis, liaison committees are in operation.

Very similar provision is made for Northern Ireland. The Department may recognise local representative committees for the area of a Board (or Boards combined) in the same professional fields with the exception of nurses and midwives but with the separation of the two ophthalmic professions (1972 Order, Art. 55). Before recognising the local committees, the Department must consult with the Board or Boards affected and with the Agency. There is also a power similar to that of the Secretary of State for Scotland to establish University Liaison Committees (Art. 21).

Relationships between central and local administration

Probably one of the least reliable indicators of the actual working relationships between central departments and local administrative bodies is the law which formally governs them. Comparison between health service provision and the personal social services (expect in Northern Ireland), however, inevitably invites discussion of their formal distinguishing characteristics in British administration.

The health service is a form of administration heavily under central control. As already indicated, ministers and departments have wide executive and supervisory powers. They have the power to define the areas, membership, constitution and, to a large extent, the functions of local Boards and Authorities. They are empowered to determine by regulation or direction their manner of working, their powers to employ staff and the terms upon which the staff are to be employed. Above all, central government has almost total control over levels of finance to be made available to Boards and Authorities (1977 Act, s. 97, 1978 Act, s.85 and 1972 Order, Art. 87), although amendments made to both the 1977 and 1978 Acts by the 1980 Act s.5 do give Health Boards and Authorities a limited right to raise money by appeals, collections, etc.

Formally the relationships between ministers and local social services/ social work authorities in England, Wales and Scotland are different. Local authorities have their areas, membership and constitution independently provided by statute (which process is, however, subject to central legislative control). Their powers too are independently conferred and they cannot readily be adjusted by central government. Ministers do, however, retain some powers of control over, for example, the appointment of chief officers (1970 Act, s.6 and 1968 Act, s.3), powers to inquire (Local Government Act 1972 and Local Government (Scotland) Act, 1973, s.210 and see also similar health service powers e.g. 1977 Act, s.84), default powers (1973 Act, s.211 and again see health service powers e.g. 1977 Act, s.85), and considerable powers of control over finance. Levels of capital expenditure are controlled (see Local

Government etc. Act 1980, Part VIII and Local Government (Scotland) Act 1973, s.94) and, through the predominance of the rate support grant in local authority recurrent expenditure, authorities have little room for manoeuvre there too.

It must nevertheless remain true that local authorities, through their separately elected membership and their independently conferred statutory powers, must enjoy an autonomy not available to health service authorities.

Bodies designed to encourage public participation

As with the local advisory and consultative bodies (B.4), the emphasis will again be upon the health service and the new bodies introduced at local level following reorganisation. The terminology varies a little, but the Community Health Councils (England and Wales), the Local Health Councils (Scotland) and the District Committees (Northern Ireland) have a common aim in encouraging participation. In Northern Ireland, of course, the Committees are relevant to the provision of personal social services as well as the health service and, to complement these, the nearest relevant bodies on the mainland, the Scottish community councils, should be mentioned. The Health Service Commissioners, Commissioners for Local Administration and the Commissioner for Complaints (as well as the Parliamentary Commissioners) are also concerned with relationships with the public and a note on these is added.

Provisions for the Community Health Councils in England and Wales is made in the 1977 Act, s.20, Schedule 7 and regulations made thereunder (see SI 1973/2217 as amended by SI 1976/791). The Secretary of State (the function is in fact delegated to Regional Authorities) is required to establish Councils (to cover the area of each Area or District Health Authority) the function of which is to represent the interests in the health service of the public in their districts and to carry out other prescribed functions. These include (SI 1973/2217) keeping the operation of the health service under review and advising the relevant Area or District Authority (which in turn is normally bound to consult Councils on proposals for substantial developments). Authorities also have a duty to supply information and to allow inspection of premises by Councils.

The membership of a Community Health Council must include at least one member appointed by each local authority in the area (and the total local authority membership must be at least half); and at least one-third of the membership drawn from voluntary organisations. No member may be a member of a Regional, Area or District Health Authority. Terms of office are normally four years and meetings must be held at least once every three months. Each Council must report annually and ensure that publicity is given to the report.

The Secretary of State has the power to establish a central body responsible for giving advice and assistance to Community Health Councils. He has set up the Association of Community Health Councils (SI 1977/1204 and SI 1977/874) for this purpose.

The Scottish equivalents of the Community Health Councils are the Local Health Councils established under the 1978 Act, s.7. This imposes an obligation upon each Health Board to submit a scheme to the Secretary of State for the establishment of local Health Councils for its area. Membership must again include local authority appointments (one-third) and representatives of other organisations (s.7 and SI 1974/2177). Functions differ only slightly from those of Community Health Councils although the annual report is made, in the first instance, to the Health Board.

Terminology is again different in Northern Ireland, but the District Committees (1972 Order, Art. 20) are designed to achieve similar purposes – but in relation to both the health and personal social services. The procedure for establishing District Committees is again by way of a scheme submitted by Board to the Department but, beyond that, the legislation is more skeletal. Requirements as to the membership of District Committees and as to their precise functions are not spelled out in the legislation although the Department has the power to issue regulations to make more detailed provision.

The Scottish community councils are not aimed specifically at either the health or personal social services. Under Part IV of the Local Government (Scotland) Act 1973, however, there has been established a pattern of (almost entirely) elected community councils whose general purpose is to ascertain, coordinate and express to the local authorities for their areas, and to public authorities, the views of the communities which they represent and to take such action in the interests of those communities as appears to be expedient and practicable. Clearly the 'local authorities' referred to include regional and islands councils in relation to their social work functions and 'public authorities' would include Health Boards.

The full powers and procedures of the 'ombudsmen' established recently to investigate complaints of injustice (or hardship) in consequence of maladministration cannot be set out here. Suffice it to say that central departments responsible for health and social services in all regions fall within the jurisdiction of the Parliamentary Commissioners (Parliamentary Commissioner Act 1967 and Parliamentary Commissioner Act (Northern Ireland) 1969); health authorities and boards fall under the Health Service Commissioners for England, Wales and Scotland (1977 Act, Part V and 1978 Act, Part VI); the Health and Social Service Boards are covered by the Commissioner for Complaints (Commissioner for Complaints Act (Northern Ireland) 1969); and English, Welsh and Scottish local authorities may by investigated by the Commissioners for Local Administration (Local Government Act 1974 and Local Government (Scotland) Act 1975).

Liaison between authorities

It is of interest to note the extent to which statutory provision is made to try to ensure integration between the health and personal social services. In a formal sense the highest degree of integration already exists, without the need for specific liaison provisions, at the level of central government. It has already been noted that, in all regions, statutory powers for health and social services are vested in a single Secretary of State or Department. The degree of integration within departments is not a matter for legal regulation. We have also noticed that, in Northern Ireland, the formal integration extends to the Health and Social Services Council, to the Central Services Agency and to the Health and Social Services Boards themselves (although the Boards are required to establish separate service committees).

The problem of liaison is primarily, therefore, one of the integration of the work of health and social services authorities at the local level in England, Wales and Scotland. There is, however, also statutory provision for cooperation in the Northern Ireland services (1972 Order, Art. 67–71). Art. 67 provides that 'in exercising their respective functions, Health and Social Services Boards, district councils, Education and Library Boards, and the Northern Ireland Housing Executive shall co-operate with one another in order to secure and advance the health and social welfare of the people of Northern Ireland'. There follow provisions for the supply of goods and services between Boards, the Agency, district councils and other bodies.

In Scotland, the 1978 Act, s.13 provides that 'in exercising their respective functions, Health Boards, local authorities and education authorities shall cooperate with one another to secure and advance the health of the people of Scotland'. S.14 requires the designation by each Health Board of a medical officer ('the designated medical officer') to carry out on behalf of local authorities *inter alia* such functions as the local authorities may, with the agreement of the Board assign to him. Powers in s.15 enable the Secretary of State, a Health Board or the Agency to supply goods and services to and permit the use of premises by local authorities. A new power under which Health Boards may make grants to local authorities towards expenditure on services of common concern was conferred by the 1980 Act, s.4.

In England and Wales, provision for cooperation is more sophisticated with the addition of the statutory requirement (1977 Act, s.22) to form joint consultative committees whose job it is to advise the health and local authorities from which they are drawn on the performance of their duties to cooperate in securing and advancing the health and welfare of the people of England and Wales. The joint committees are formed by Area Authorities and the local authorities within their areas with a membership agreed between all authorities concerned (s.22 and SI 1974/190). There is further provision for health authorities to make available to local authorities goods, services and facilities and to make grants (1977 Act, ss. 26–28 as amended by the 1980 Act, s.3–4); and local authorities (by amendment to the Local Government Act 1972, s.113) are able to place their officers at the disposal of Regional and Area Health Authorities and vice versa (NHS Reorganisation Act 1973, Schedule 4, para 151).

5 Patterns of Organisation for Health: a systems overview of the National Service in the United Kingdom

David Hunter

Introduction

If observers of the National Health Service (NHS) are aware of the existence of four health services in the United Kingdom (in England, Wales, Scotland and Northern Ireland), rather than just one, the fact is usually only fleetingly acknowledged if at all. The practice in much of the literature is to centre discussion on the English Health Service which is deemed typical of arrangements elsewhere in the UK.[1] While it is reasonable to assume that many of the insights derived from studies of the English Health Service also apply to the NHS in Wales, Scotland and Northern Ireland, the *extent* of the similarities, and differences, remains to be explored.

The focus of this chapter is on *inter-nation* differences within the UK as distinct from *intra-nation* ones. The exclusion of the intra-nation dimension is not intended to diminish its importance. On the contrary, heterogeneity *within* each of the four nations of the UK is as, perhaps more, prevalent as that *between* them. This point is pursued a little further in the next section. But a primary focus on inter-nation differences is justified because of the lack of attention they have received from researchers and policy analysts. In contrast, studies of intra-nation variations are undertaken from time to time, especially in England.[2] While there is some published work on the Scottish Health Service,[3] there appears to be no published analytical work on the NHS in Wales or Northern Ireland. However, although there is scope for further work of this kind, the inter-nation dimension has been neglected altogether. It is hard to avoid the impression that the reasons for a lack of a comparative focus in regard to the NHS in the UK have less to do with the view that there is little to be gained from such an exercise, and much more to do with the general gravitation in British public administration, or policy analysis, research towards the 'centre', that is, London, Westminster, Whitehall, the Department of Health and Social Security or whatever.

That all four health services share common purposes and a number of features, as well as having some problems in common, is beyond doubt.

But by overlooking, or blurring, whether through ignorance or for convenience, the variations that *are* present, much of potential interest in the study of social policy and the development of organisations and services escapes analysis. Because variations go unexplored (assuming, that is, that they have been identified in the first place), it becomes all too easy misleadingly to assume that there is really only one NHS, namely, that administered from the DHSS in London. Practices elsewhere in the UK are perceived, if at all, as deviations from this model rather than as separate, or modified, responses to specific circumstances prevailing in countries with marginally different socio-political (and geopolitical) environments. Despite the spate of nationalist fervour for much of the 1970s, which has abated for the time being, both Wales and Scotland remain wedded to the Westminster/Whitehall political axis, while continuing to enjoy varying degrees of administrative devolution. Northern Ireland, on the other hand, has been wracked by religious and political turbulence since the Reformation in the sixteenth century, a fact which sets it apart from the rest of the UK. As Rose has argued, 'Northern Ireland has always been governed without consensus. Less than half the population has been *fully allegiant*, that is, prepared to support the constitutional government of the day and to comply with its basic laws.'[4] From 1921 until 1972, a system of home rule prevailed in Northern Ireland based at Stormont which was notable for the considerable degree of executive and legislative autonomy it possessed. The revival of the disturbances in Northern Ireland in 1969 led, in 1972, to the suspension of Stormont and the start of direct rule from Westminster. The government of the Province is presently the responsibility of the Secretary of State for Northern Ireland, and the Northern Ireland Office over which he presides is the counterpart of the Welsh and Scottish Offices.

The purpose of this chapter is to consider some of the key organisational features of the four health services operating in the UK and, in so doing, to highlight the chief differences between them. Where possible, given the existing state of knowledge, the likely significance of these differences for policy-making, implementation, and policy outcomes is briefly considered. Their significance for comparative research within the UK is also touched upon.

Comparative studies

Comparative studies of public policy have generally taken one of two directions. The first has been to study a limited number of comparable political systems and a limited range of policy areas.[5] Because of the limited focus of these studies, their ability to produce meaningful generalisations is severely constrained. The second approach seeks greater cross-national generalisations by examining a much larger number and variety of nations in terms of aggregate data. But while breadth is achieved, depth is sacrificed and much of the rich detail underlying the development of public policies is lost. Ideally, what is required is a synthesis of the two approaches – a combination of multi-nation studies and analyses of specific case studies conducted in selected policy fields. A recent example of such an approach is Leichter's comparative study of health care policy in four nations.[6] But even this middle way has drawbacks. As in all cross-national studies of health care policy which include the UK,[7] the NHS is treated as a uniform, monolithic entity and intra–UK variations are simply discounted, or ignored altogether. Therefore, there are gaps in the interstices of comparative policy analysis in the health field (and probably in other fields too) which merit attention if a fuller understanding of public policy is sought. Comparative studies within the UK, although not strictly cross-national, ought not to be regarded as insular and parochial, but rather as supplementing other types of comparative study that are truly cross-national and macro in approach.

The comparative study of health care policy should take account of the broad social and economic forces which assist in determining health status among social classes and the type, and use made, of services provided. But this macro approach needs to be balanced by micro studies of how services operate and how decisions get taken, employing what Martin calls 'very fine brushstrokes' (see Chapter 3 of this volume). Comparative research of this type remains undeveloped within the UK. Yet in a setting where broadly similar social and economic conditions prevail between the four countries, despite some important differences in detail, the opportunities to engage in micro studies are potentially attractive. Advocating comparative work of an intra-UK variety does not preclude studies which seek to compare, say, Scotland with similar countries in Europe like Norway and Finland. There is scope for a wide variety of studies each with its own particular set of aims.

As has been implied, comparing intra-UK health services presents different problems from those encountered in more familiar comparative studies of health systems. For a start, many of the major concerns of cross-national studies, whether of an aggregate data type or of the case study variety, are simply irrelevant in a study of health services in the UK. In terms of ideology, models of welfare, finance and basic organisational structure, there are no grounds for comparison (see Chapter 2 of this volume). The differences that exist are of a different order. Moreover, they are often partially hidden amidst the minutiae of management arrangements as these have evolved in each of the four countries, and they are most unlikely to be detected by a macro-scan of the NHS in the UK which, in any case, would probably be concerned with rather more fundamental matters. However, in terms of the debate over health policy in the UK, these marginal differences, which may reflect deeper, and quite significant, political, economic and cultural schisms, may be important. Moreover, there may be an intrinsic interest in accounting for the seeming paradox of system differences proliferating in a unitary state (i.e. the UK) which has been described as 'the most centralised of all Western industrialised democracies'.[8]

Context

Broad contextual features of intra-UK health services generally receive scant attention. For instance, it is not widely known that in addition to sometimes striking differences in resource provision within each of the four parts of the UK, such differences also occur *between* them.[9] In terms of per capita expenditure of health services and on numbers of staff, some parts of the UK fare considerably better than others. Wales, Scotland and Northern Ireland receive a larger proportion of expenditure on health than England. As Table 5.1 shows, per capita expenditure on health services in Scotland in 1976/7 was 21.2% higher than that in England and 18.4% higher than in Wales.[10] Northern Ireland was higher still but has a lower doctor/population ratio than Scotland which, in the distribution of health manpower, comes out on top in the UK. In Scotland, as Table 5.2 shows, there are over 15 doctors per 10,000 population compared with 11.43 for the UK as a whole, and a lower average number of patients with each GP.[11] There is also a more generous provision of nurse manpower. Within England, as can be seen from Table 5.1, per capita expenditure is higher in the four Thames regions which cover London and the South-East of England than in the other regions, although it still falls below expenditure in Scotland and Northern Ireland.

These figures on expenditure and manpower make no allowance for differences in demand or need for health services, nor for differences in the cost of delivering health care, although these factors have been cited to account, in large part, for Scotland's generous share of resources (and much the same applies to Northern Ireland and, to a lesser extent, Wales where there are, like Scotland, a few dense urban areas, many with declining heavy industries, and large tracts of sparsely populated rural hinterlands and, especially in Scotland's case, islands). Moreover, demographic patterns affect resource distribution and access to services. Here, the four parts of the UK display small, but significant, differences:

Table 5.1 Distribution of health expenditure, UK 1976/7

£ per capita

	Hospital services expenditure	*Community health and family practitioner services expenditure*	*Total expenditure*[a]
England	61.76	28.31	104.88
Northern	56.19	28.42	100.13
Yorkshire	56.86	27.42	97.44
Trent	50.49	26.67	93.80
East Anglia	53.83	26.94	95.22
NW Thames	74.91	33.21	122.38
NE Thames	76.35	25.95	117.00
SE Thames	73.61	29.28	118.17
SW Thames	67.00	28.67	112.73
Wessex	52.44	28.15	94.00
Oxford	53.18	28.23	96.09
South Western	57.87	30.50	103.33
West Midlands	52.65	26.96	91.52
Mersey	62.16	27.92	107.16
North Western	57.63	28.88	100.46
Wales	61.50	31.21	107.39
Scotland	78.10	30.00	127.10
N. Ireland	83.07	33.67	138.67
United Kingdom	63.84	28.76	107.98

Source: Compiled from Central Statistical Office, *Regional Statistics*, Vol. 14, London, HMSO, 1979. Cited in Royal Commission on the NHS[9].

Note: [a]Includes 'headquarters administration', 'other services' and capital expenditure not shown separately.

Scotland and Northern Ireland have slightly younger populations than the population of England. The figures are in Table 5.3.

Despite a healthier resource situation in Wales, Scotland and Northern Ireland, this is not reflected in mortality rates where the three countries continue to lag behind England as a whole (see Table 5.4). The discrepancy between available resources and mortality rates is particularly marked in Scotland. A breakdown of England into its regions, as shown in Table 5.4, reveals that several of them, North Western in particular, have similar, or even slightly higher, mortality rates than those prevailing in the rest of the UK. In the case of these regions, their resource position is not as buoyant as that outside England. Of course, there are also resource imbalances *within* Wales, Scotland and Northern Ireland and although they may not be as marked as those among the English regions, they are nevertheless of some concern to policy-makers and others in the three countries.

Table 5.2 Distribution of health manpower, UK 1977

per 10,000 population

	General medical practitioners	*Hospital doctors (wte)*[a]	*General dental practitioners*	*Nurses and midwives (wte)*
England	4.84	6.13	2.55	73.5
Northern	4.55	6.24	1.84	71.4
Yorkshire	4.70	5.62	2.18	73.6
Trent	4.54	5.14	1.88	66.1
East Anglia	4.85	5.71	2.20	65.6
NW Thames	5.48	7.84	4.01	75.4
NE Thames	5.10	7.40	2.77	76.6
SE Thames	5.01	6.85	2.91	80.5
SW Thames	5.17	6.25	3.61	76.5
Wessex	4.98	5.45	2.72	68.5
Oxford	4.73	6.04	2.51	62.3
South Western	5.17	5.32	2.97	74.7
West Midlands	4.56	5.45	2.10	67.9
Mersey	4.60	6.13	2.44	80.6
North Western	4.55	6.59	2.12	75.0
Wales	5.05	5.96	2.09	79.0
Scotland	5.98	9.19	2.33	102.2
N. Ireland	5.56	7.84	2.27	98.6
United Kingdom	4.98	6.45	2.50	77.1

Source: Royal Commission on the NHS[9]

Notes: [a]Whole time equivalents.
Figures for English regions are for 1978.

Table 5.3 Population structure, 1977

	% of population aged 0–14	*% of population aged 65+*
England	22.2	14.4
Scotland	23.1	13.5
N. Ireland	26.7	13.3

Source: *Social Trends No. 9*

Trying to make sense of these discrepancies is not easy. The Royal Commission on the NHS observed that 'in 1977 Scotland, with 50% more hospital doctors and about 40% more nurses and midwives per 10,000 population than England, nonetheless had a comparatively lower life expectancy and a higher infant mortality rate'.[12] The Report contrasted these facts to the situation in the Trent region of England,

Table 5.4 Mortality rates, UK 1977[a]

	Infant mortality rate	*Perinatal mortality rate*	*Standardised mortality ratio[b]*	
			M	*F*
England	13.7	16.9	99	99
Northern	14.9	19.1	111	109
Yorkshire	15.5	18.1	105	105
Trent	13.9	16.7	103	102
East Anglia	11.2	13.0	89	96
NW Thames	11.8	14.8	89	90
NE Thames	14.0	16.1	94	92
SE Thames	13.1	16.8	95	92
SW Thames	11.6	14.6	90	95
Wessex	13.1	15.5	92	92
Oxford	12.7	15.0	90	96
South Western	12.5	16.2	93	97
West Midlands	15.0	19.4	103	103
Mersey	14.4	18.8	110	109
North Western	14.8	18.5	113	111
Wales	13.5	17.9	108	106
Scotland	16.1	18.3	112	109
N. Ireland	17.2	21.1	112	115

Source: Office of Population Censuses and Surveys. Cited in Royal Commission on the NHS[9].

Notes: [a]The infant mortality rate is the number of deaths under one year of age per 1000 live births; the perinatal mortality rate is the number of deaths occurring after the twenty-eighth week of pregnancy or during the first week of life per 1000 total births; and the standardised mortality ratio (SMR) compares the number of deaths actually occurring in an area with those which would be expected if national mortality rates by age and sex were applicable to the population of that area.

[b]England, English regions and Wales based on England and Wales = 100. Scotland and Northern Ireland based on UK = 100.

until recently 'generally regarded as being the most under-funded regional health authority', with a standardised mortality ratio close to the average for England. The only conclusion to be drawn is that 'the relationship between health service resources and the health of the population served, as measured by mortality rates, is far from simple. . . .'[13]

Godber maintains that in England there has been 'so much smaller provision made [for health services] than in Scotland, that it has not been possible to provide the extra money needed' for deprived areas in the Midlands and the North of England.[14] The advocacy role of the Scottish Office (in particular the Scottish Home and Health Department

(SHHD) which is responsible for the NHS in Scotland), the Northern Ireland Office (in particular the Department of Health and Social Services (DHSS (NI)) and, to a lesser extent, the Welsh Office (considerably younger than the Scottish Office, having been created in 1964 with fewer powers), which enables these countries to exploit whatever opportunity there is within the central financing arrangements, ought, in Godber's opinion, to be applied to the areas where there are the greatest deficiencies in England. 'The example of Scotland in securing a large and increasing advantage in funds and manpower and the more recent relative gain by Wales shows how the urgent needs of other regions, which have no separate line of approach to central funds, can fail to obtain recognition'.[15] No empirical data are available which either support, or refute, Godber's analysis based, as it probably is, on his experience as former Chief Medical Officer (1960–73) in the DHSS in England. But Godber is not alone in his conviction that the separate political voices of Wales, Scotland and Northern Ireland (in the specific shape of the respective Secretaries of State who are full members of the Cabinet) have given these countries a special advantage which they have maintained when questions of resource allocation are being decided.[16]

The Resource Allocation Working Party (RAWP) policy,[17] which has counterparts in the other three countries,[18] is designed to correct regional imbalances in England, but progress is slow at a time of low growth. Moreover, the policy is dependent upon political will in London for its success and it is possible that it is being pursued less vigorously by the present Conservative administration.[19] However, RAWP (and its counterparts) only apply within each country and while it may be laudable to try and remove resource imbalances occurring within each of the four countries, no attempt has been made to tackle the inter-nation basis of resource allocation which is Godber's chief concern. Politically such a move seems remote. Commenting on the absence of any attempt to equalise health care resources between the UK countries, Maynard and Ludbrook point out that 'the application of the RAWP formula to the UK shows that Scotland and Northern Ireland are over-funded relative to England and Wales and that any policy of allocating resources equally across the UK, rather than within each part of the UK, would result in the NHS budgets of Scotland and Northern Ireland being reduced substantially'.[20] If there were one genuinely national (in UK terms) health service, instead of four services, resource imbalances on such a scale would not exist. A further problem with resource allocation formulae is that they have not always succeeded in altering allocations at local level.[21]

In essence, the differences between the four constituent parts of the UK in the provision of health care lie in the area of administration and institutional arrangements which reflect, to some extent, different historical traditions and political trends. Differences in policy, where these occur, have been more subtle. This is not to suggest that all policy pronouncements emanate, however indirectly, from London. While it is true that the Whitehall departments in London initiate much of the policy common to the UK, considerable divergences are possible and, indeed, do occur. Moreover, there are occasions when the policy lead is taken in UK countries besides England. For instance, in Scotland and Northern Ireland health centres for general practice services have expanded more rapidly than in England which is only now increasing their number. At the end of 1979, 54% of all GPs practised from health centres in Northern Ireland. Although other examples can be cited, one further policy difference merits a brief mention. The English policy of reducing beds for mental illness and providing alternative care in the community has never been explicitly adopted in Scotland, although there has been a fall in the number of available staffed beds. As in England, there is a desire in Scotland to see a community based service evolve; the essential difference between the two countries lies in the fact that in Scotland it is believed that developing the community care services should be done while maintaining the mental hospitals as part of the network. The English notion that these hospitals should be closed, a policy which the Royal Commission claims is unrealistic[22] and which is resisted by the professions involved, has never been accepted.

While it is often asserted, generally correctly, that UK health policy originates in London, the 'traffic flow' is not always that simple. This raises the nature of central-local relations within the NHS in the UK, not only as these operate within each country, but also as they operate between the DHSS in England and the Welsh Office, the SHHD and the DHSS (NI). There are, therefore, two separate sets of central-local relations about which there remains considerable ignorance. These relations are compounded by trying to pinpoint where policy-making begins and ends and where implementation takes over. It is now recognised that it is not possible to make a simple division between the two activities, spatially or in any other way. In reality they are much more blurred.[23]

One other contextual factor of some importance in intra-UK health care provision should be mentioned, namely, the private health care sector and its relationship with the NHS. The most significant aspect of this is its variable impact throughout the UK. Private practice in NHS hospitals (i.e. pay-beds) is concentrated in London and the South-East, and in larger conurbations in the West Midlands (Birmingham) and North-West (Manchester) of England. Elsewhere in the UK it is of marginal importance. Nevertheless, the subject is of mounting interest in the context of the English Health Service. The last two years or so have witnessed a steady expansion of the private health sector.[24] Major shifts in the balance of care between the public and private sectors could occur. The Government is also intent upon fostering closer relations between the two sectors and set up an interdepartmental working party to study alternative finance. These developments are bound to have an impact on the NHS which could be greater than that arising from the pay-beds controversy in 1976 which soured relations between service providers.[25] The almost total absence of private practice outside England may account, in part, for a working atmosphere among service providers that is less charged politically. If, as the Royal Commission concluded, 'the main importance of pay beds (for the NHS) lies in the passions aroused and the consequential dislocation of work which then occurs',[26] one can only speculate upon what might be the consequences of current developments for the NHS in each of the four countries. It is necessary, however, to keep a sense of perspective. Private practice is not widespread in England but is confined to London, to Manchester and to Birmingham. There is a tendency for London-centred problems to set, and dominate, the UK health policy agenda which can be misleading.

Contextual features, such as those just mentioned, are noteworthy in so far as they assist in shaping the climate in which health services are administered and delivered, and in accounting for many of the differences that exist between the constituent parts of the UK.

Foci for comparison

What follows is not a comprehensive review of the NHS in the UK but a selection of what appear to be some of the more significant variations in system design and in the operation (perhaps performance too, although, as explained later, this is harder to determine) of the NHS in an intra-UK context. These variations are considered within a framework comprising the key themes running through all four health services when they were first reorganised in 1973 (Northern Ireland) and 1974 (England, Wales and Scotland), and then again in 1982.

There are three main overlapping themes although it is appropriate for analytical purposes to consider them separately. They are (i) *integration* (the unification of the pre-1974 tripartite structure); (ii) *management* (including notions of efficiency and effectiveness); and (iii) *planning* (including priority-setting and resource-allocation procedures). Within each theme, it is useful to distinguish between differences in *structure* (organisational arrangements) and *process* (the actual operation of the arrangements). A third category might also be included, *output* (the nature, and impact, of services that are provided), but this is more problematic since there is a lack of reliable knowledge. Nevertheless, a satisfactory analysis of output is dependent to some degree upon a thorough examination of structure and process. While it is simple enough to chart structural variations between health services in the UK, there is greater difficulty in examining processes both within, and more especially between, intra-UK services. Consequently there is considerable ignorance about them and about the interaction of all three elements: structure, process and output.

The perspective adopted here, with its focus on three themes, is sufficiently broad to embrace a range of specific issues, including: centre-periphery relations (on two levels); periphery-periphery relations, especially those between health and personal social services; relations between various parts of the health service in each country; priority-setting; and policy implementation.

Subsequent sections endeavour to show how each health service in the UK has responded to each of the themes listed above, and to indicate where, and in what ways, the response has differed between services. These themes were not only instrumental in shaping the arrangements which emerged in the early 1970s, but are important if an understanding of how the four services are operating is sought. This remains the case despite the fact that the NHS throughout the UK has recently undergone further structural reform. A fourth theme, participation by providers and consumers, has been omitted since similar participatory mechanisms operate throughout the UK with no discernible differences.

Briefly, the recent changes are intended to simplify the administration of the NHS and to reduce central interference in the affairs of local health authorities by granting local decision-makers greater discretionary powers.[27] In December 1979, the Government published three consultative documents on structural and management issues covering England and Wales,[28], Scotland[29] and Northern Ireland[30] respectively. These were loosely derived from the report of the Royal Commission on the NHS which appeared in July 1979. More important were the proposals which Ministers, in particular Patrick Jenkin, Secretary of State for Social Services, 1979–81, and Gerard Vaughan, Minister for Health, 1979–82, had formulated while in opposition. Although the consultation period was straightforward in England and, to a lesser extent, in Scotland, it was a protracted affair in Wales and Northern Ireland, Partly for these reasons, different timetables have been followed in each country in regard to the completion of reforms.

Ironically, given the magnitude of the changes proposed, progress has been most rapid in England. The English circular[31] announcing Government plans was the first to appear. Major changes included the abolition of Area Health Authorities (AHAs) and the creation of District Health Authorities (DHAs), an emphasis on unit management, and changes in functional management. Regional Health Authorities (RHAs) were entrusted with the task of drawing up plans for the new DHAs. At a later stage, once the new structure is in place, the regions themselves may be reviewed. The new DHAs took over on 1 April 1982 and they, together with the RHAs, have been determining appropriate management arrangements below district level. Most DHAs have populations of between 200,000 and 400,000; about twenty have populations below 150,000 and seven exceed 500,000. Single-district areas have been subjected to minimal turbulence.

The Scottish circular[32] appeared in March 1981 and its main proposals were for a phasing out of districts in multi-district areas, of which there are ten, a stress on unit management and changes in functional management. Unlike England, no changes in statutory authorities have occurred. The proposed changes were to be undertaken by the health boards with minimal involvement by the SHHD and were, if possible, to be completed by April 1982, altough the timetable is flexible.

Although in Wales, and especially in Northern Ireland, the opportunity has been taken to review a range of issues which has been giving cause for concern since the 1974 (1973 in Northern Ireland) reorganisation of the NHS,[33] only limited changes have in fact occurred. In Wales, the relevant circular appeared in June 1981.[34] The AHAs have been retained (they resemble English DHAs in population terms) and the districts abolished. The only statutory change is that one of the AHAs has been divided, thus creating a new AHA and bringing the total to nine. In Northern Ireland a circular[35] on the NHS appeared in June 1981. Like Scotland and Wales, existing statutory authorities have been retained and districts have been abolished. A number of important changes were proposed in regard to the composition of area management teams (mentioned below) and to unit management. The changes were to be implemented by the end of March 1983.

Given the modest, though not unimportant, nature of the changes taking place outside England, it seems reasonable to conclude that nothing would have changed in Scotland, Wales and Northern Ireland had it not been for Ministers' determination to simplify the arrangements in England. This is not to disregard, or minimise, the various changes but it is an exaggeration to perceive these as constituting major restructuring. The changes in all four countries are designed to alter practices within intra-UK services and should not affect relations between the four services. At appropriate points, the new changes, and their likely consequences, are referred to in the sections which follow.

Integration

The reorganisation of the NHS in the constituent parts of the UK in 1973 and 1974 was chiefly about integration which, above all, entailed replacing the tripartite structure which had existed since 1948 when the NHS was created. This model had denied, or at best impeded, any continuity between primary, hospital and community care since these services were organised under separate authorities. The 1982 reorganisation remains committed to the notion of integration, although certain changes seem to mark a retreat from this. These are considered below.

It is useful to distinguish between *structural* integration, involving organisational factors, and *process* integration, involving behavioural and attitudinal factors, because while on an organisation chart integration has occurred in varying degrees throughout the UK, it is not so easy to determine the impact of this on professional attitudes or on collaborative practices between professional groups both within the NHS and between health and related services.

It has been argued that such integration as has occurred is integration of 'narrowly conceived medical care and not *other* forms of care that are available through other agencies'.[36] Reorganisation of the NHS in the 1970s did not encompass the roles of, among others, the Departments of Employment, Education and Science nor, with the exception of Northern Ireland, Social Services Departments (SSDs), and consequently produced a new set of 'frontier', or coordination, problems. In England, Wales and Scotland local authority SSDs (social work departments in Scotland) remain separate from the NHS as do housing and environmental activities in all four countries.

If integration, as the term has been applied to health services, is viewed as a continuum, with Northern Ireland at one extreme representing the maximum degree of integration (structurally and possibly in process terms too) that currently exists in the UK, and England, Wales and Scotland positioned at various points along the continuum towards the opposite extreme of minimal integration, then the variations that exist can be more easily observed.

In Northern Ireland, not only have health services been brought together, but also personal social services have been merged with health. Integration on this scale, and across services, seems to have been possible to achieve for three reasons: (i) Seebohm-type SSDs[37] had been in existence in Northern Ireland since 1948 which meant that the professions in this field were not undergoing reorganisation along the lines of personal social services (PSS) in England and Wales (Scottish arrangements in social work differ from those in England and Wales in some significant ways and were in advance of these two countries); (ii) reform of the health service was closely related to the reform of local government which was not the case elsewhere in the UK; the Review Body on Local Government, which reported in 1970, endorsed the proposal to integrate the two services; and (iii) because, it is alleged, social workers were more secure in their status as professionals, they were less defensive than social workers in the UK in their attitudes towards the medical profession. This last point should not be overstated. In Northern Ireland, as elsewhere, health services are more integrated than health *and* PSS where barriers remain, even if they are somewhat less pronounced than those that existed previously. Some social workers *were* apprehensive about medical domination and to placate them separate social services committees operate within each of the four health and social services boards. These committees are the equivalent of the health services committees which provide a forum for the medical profession. In addition, until 1979, there was an earmarked budget for certain PSS in order to safeguard them.

Developments in Northern Ireland are in marked contrast to those elsewhere in the UK where *coordination* between health and PSS has been stressed rather than *integration*. Nevertheless, there are important differences among the three countries as well as between them and Northern Ireland. In England and Wales, Joint Consultative Committees have been created made up of health and local authority representatives. An extension of this arrangement has been the establishment of Joint Care Planning Teams and the introduction of joint finance, the purpose of which is to facilitate joint planning between health and local authorities. The arrangements allow the two sets of authorities to contribute jointly, in agreed proportions, to the capital and revenue costs of schemes, the cost of which would normally fall wholly upon local authorities. The health authorities' revenue contribution extends only over a limited period of years, at the end of which the local authority has to carry the full running costs. Understandably, and especially at a time of financial uncertainty and spending cuts, many local authorities are wary of entering into such agreements with health authorities since they are a commitment on the authorities' future resources.

In Scotland a more flexible approach to collaboration was adopted initially. The White Paper on reorganisation merely stated that 'the machinery for fostering close working relationships need not be specified in legislation in precise terms . . . .'[38] However, various working parties and sub-groups kept the subject under review since 1971 and changes in existing liaison machinery were recommended in the report of the last working party.[39] The report's main recommendation was that formal machinery should be set up in the shape of Joint Liaison Committees, but there was no mention at this stage of introducing joint financing to underpin collaborative activities. Nevertheless, mounting pressure for an initiative similar to that operating in England and Wales was successful, for the Health Services Act 1980 extends the scheme to Scotland where it is known as support finance.

A key feature of the recent reforms of the NHS in England, as already mentioned, is the removal of the area tier. Area Health Authorities (AHAs) were created primarily to forge a link with local government and in most cases their boundaries matched the areas served by local authorities responsible for social services (i.e. the counties, districts within the six metropolitan counties and the London boroughs) of which there are 106. The principle of coterminosity is no longer held to be sacrosanct (it no longer exists in about half the areas) and, despite belated concern on the Government's part, it seems clear that collaboration will now be more difficult.[40] Government concern has manifested itself in repeated calls for collaboration to be given priority by the new DHAs culminating in a circular and, more forcibly, in the publication of suggestions for transferring resources from the NHS to local government to overcome some of the drawbacks arising from joint finance.[41] There are to date no plans for resource transfers elsewhere in the UK. Significantly, in Wales and Scotland the principle of coterminosity has been preserved with the retention of the area tier, although the reason for this is not clear. About three-quarters of DHAs in England fall within the population band 100,000 to 300,000 compared with only one-quarter of Scottish health boards. Yet, nearly three-quarters of the existing Scottish districts are within the population band 100,000 to 300,000 (i.e. like the English DHAs). But districts in Scotland do not form the basis of the modified Scottish Health Service. It does appear that a difference of principle underlies the reform in England and that less weight has been attached to the principle of coterminosity and more to the desire for smaller authorities. Although there have been demands in both Wales and Scotland for a re-examination of area boundaries, these, with one exception in Wales, have been rejected.

Integration at national level in each of the four countries varies just as it does at sub-national level. In England, Wales and Northern Ireland, the central departments – DHSS, Welsh Office (Health and Social Work Department) and DHSS (NI) – are organised on a more integrated basis in terms of strategic policy formation between health and PSS than is the case in Scotland where the Scottish Office, and two of its departments, are charged with important policy-making and executive functions in these spheres. The Scottish Office is divided into five depattments, one of which, the Scottish Education Department (SED), carries out the functions exercised by the Department of Education and Science in England, with the major exception that certain functions associated with PSS (the responsibility of the DHSS in England) are exercised by the

Social Work Services Group in the SED. Although local government in England comes under the Department of the Environment, the Secretary of State for Social Services has responsibility for guiding PSS. In Scotland, while the Secretary of State is in overall charge of several other functions besides health, each of which is the responsibility of a separate Minister in England, this element of 'corporateness' (which is also a feature of the 'top of the office' in Northern Ireland and Wales) does not overcome the fact that in both these countries, and in England, integration at central level is devoid of the more obvious departmental barriers that survive in Scotland. In confirmation of this, with the exception of Scotland, the various priorities documents that have appeared review health and PSS jointly.[42] Significantly, the two Scottish documents[43] confine themselves to the NHS. In an attempt partially to overcome this institutionalised division, since 1979 the Scottish Parliamentary Under-Secretary of State for Health has also been responsible for social work services in Scotland.

The above account of integration has, unavoidably, grossly simplified what, in reality, amounts to a complex pattern of interaction at central level both within, and between, the four countries. Its effect on policy-making remains to be explored more fully. For instance, it may be that the Scottish arrangements, with their predominantly departmental bias despite the existence of the Secretary of State who has coordinating responsibilities which are, in theory, much wider than those of any of his Whitehall colleagues in England, are more, or less, effective in fostering collaboration between interrelated services than practices elsewhere in the UK. Wiseman, in a study of collaboration between the Social Work Services Group and the SHHD, argues that 'the nature of the impediments to collaboration . . . indicates that bringing together' the two departments within one department of the Scottish Office 'would not be the panacea that many seem to believe'.[44]

Despite the termination of the tripartite structure of the NHS which, for the most part, has signalled the demise of formal segregation, there remains in the organisation of primary care services in England and Wales an element of formal separation. In both countries, Family Practitioner Committees (FPCs) were established in 1974 to look after the interests of GPs. They had an independent status from AHAs to which they were attached until April 1982. Such an arrangement allegedly caused difficulties for AHAs entrusted with the planning and development of integrated health services, including health centres. The Government has retained FPCs but changes in their status will occur, although these could take five years. It has been decided that FPCs are to become separate health authorities funded directly by the DHSS. Meantime, the ninety FPCs in England which matched AHA boundaries will be linked to nominated DHAs as a temporary measure. These changes are bound to reinforce the reclusive nature of FPC activities which is inappropriate for planning purposes. If general practitioners regard FPCs as an essential safeguard for their independence then their absence in Scotland and Northern Ireland surely dispels this illusion. Structurally, at any rate, the integration of primary care services with hospital and community care services has gone further in both countries. In Scotland, in place of FPCs, committees of the area health boards look after the interests of GPs. In Northern Ireland, GPs contract to the four field authorities, but the Central Services Agency (see sub-section on management below) has a strong role in the administration of GP services. Improved integration between GPs and other health services may be assisted by the decision to enlarge area executive teams to include a representative of GPs in the area.[45] There is a large measure of agreement throughout the UK that some of the difficulties in primary care arise from the contractual status of GPs but it may be significant that the Royal Commission on the NHS should conclude that the absence in Scotland and Northern Ireland of separate machinery for administering GP services 'assists the integrated planning of health services'.[46] On the strength of this the Commission recommends the adoption in England and Wales of the practice in Scotland. However, as already mentioned, the Government has chosen to pursue a different course.

Despite the Commission's conviction, it is frequently alleged that the more integrative arrangements prevailing in Scotland and Northern Ireland are, in fact, of marginal importance. For instance, Kogan *et al.* conclude from their field interview survey that integration of GP services in these two countries had not made any substantial difference to the involvement of GPs in general health service management. However, at the researchers' own admission, they were unable in the time available to treat their data to deeper analysis and verification. Moreover, most of the team's research was undertaken in England where three authorities were investigated as compared with one authority in each of the three remaining countries.[47]

Apart from the variations cited above, and others which have not been mentioned, where there are clear structural differences in the approach to integration adopted by all four countries, there are other less visible features present about which little is known. While these may be partly responsible for the precise structural arrangements that have evolved in each country, it is also possible that they account for the way in which these arrangements actually operate. Numerous socio-political, and medico-political, factors of varying potency are at play within each country (some were noted earlier) all of which have a bearing on the achievement of genuine, as distinct from symbolic, integration both within, and between, services. It is extremely likely that such legacies have some effect on policy-making, on priorities and on the biases present with a country's health service. They might, for instance, help to explain the high expenditure on the hospital service in Scotland and conversely, the more rapid development of PSS in England.

The question of scale (the assumption invariably being that small *is* beautiful) crops up in all comparisons between England and the other three countries and yet there is no conclusive evidence, other than of an anecdotal variety, one way or the other.[48] It is frequently argued that because the sub-national administrative units in Wales, Scotland and Northern Ireland are smaller, and hence perhaps more manageable, than in England this facilitates communication between tiers, and between them and the central departments. But how far is this so? While informal relations may flourish in the three smaller countries, it may also be possible for the centre to intervene more readily in the affairs of health authorities, thereby reducing their discretion and room for manoeuvre and, ironically, making for greater centralisation than exists in England. This point is taken up again in the next sub-section.

Management

A commitment to better, more rational, management through improved efficiency and effectiveness in resource use was a core theme of the NHS reorganisation in the 1970s, despite the fact that the structures which finally emerged in each of the four countries owed as much, perhaps more, to political compromise as to pure management theory.[49] Moreover, the emphasis on management was not uniform throughout the UK. Whereas in England, Wales and Northern Ireland details of the respective management structures were worked out by each central department with assistance from teams of management consultants,[50] in Scotland the arrangements emerged internally within the SHHD. Unlike the rest of the UK, no report concerned specifically with management structures was commissioned. General principles were enunciated through a series of circulars but the details of structures below area level were left to the area boards to work out and refer to the Secretary of State for approval. This detached departmental pose can be contrasted with the attempt at precision and clarity elsewhere in the UK. Nevertheless, it would be surprising if civil servants in the SHHD had not been influenced to some extent by what was happening in the other parts of the UK, especially in England, i.e. the 'spill-over effect'. Their thinking was also heavily influenced by a report on administrative practice in Scottish hospital boards published in 1966.[51] The report had aroused interest in England prior to reorganisation and, conceivably, had an impact on the thinking of officials in the DHSS as they reflected upon the future shape of the English Health Service. Certainly, the Farquharson–Lang report contains much of the managerial style and quest for greater efficiency and effectiveness which merged forcefully as central themes in the reorganised NHS.[52] Although improved management remains a feature of the latest round of reorganisation, its focus has shifted. During the first restructuring of the Service, attention was lavished on regions, areas and districts. Now, there is a stress on units of management below districts since it is the Government's view, one shared by many within the Service, that this important level was neglected in the early 1970s. It is also anticipated that 'better' management will result from the demise of areas in England (and districts elsewhere).

Most of the changes in the NHS resulting from the two reorganisations have occurred at sub-national level. The most obvious structural difference in the NHS in the UK is the presence of a regional tier in England which is not a feature of the other three systems, although, prior to reorganisation, both Wales and Scotland were divided into regions. Functions performed by regions in England are divided between central departments and special agencies in Wales, Scotland and Northern Ireland. The Welsh Health Technical Services Organisation, the Common Services Agency in Scotland and the Central Services Agency in Northern Ireland are organised jointly by the health authorities and central departments in the respective countries. The agencies provide a range of technical support services, the mix varying in each country.

The role of the central department in England is very different from the role of its counterparts in the other three countries where there is no regional tier. Central departments in Wales, Scotland and Northern Ireland have a dual function: to perform the usual duties required of a government department and, in addition, to assume responsibility for managing health services. The problem of central interference in the NHS is perceived by many to be a real one. In Wales and Northern Ireland, for instance, the 1982 reforms of the NHS have been seen by many within the NHS as providing an opportunity to press for a regional authority in both countries which would be interposed between the central department and the health service.

Predictably, the Government has ruled out such a solution to the problem of separating the central department's regional (and managerial) responsibilities from its political and governmental responsibilities. It has been argued in Wales[53] and Northern Ireland[54] that a regional authority would overlap with the work of the central department and that this would be unavoidable if the Secretary of State was to fulfil his responsibilities to Parliament. In Wales, according to the Welsh Office, this was a compelling reason for not continuing the Welsh Hospital Board after 1974 since a one-to-one relationship did not work well. A regional organisation is also ruled out for Scotland[55] where five regions existed until 1974. Paradoxically, while Scotland, and particularly Wales and Northern Ireland, ponder over whether a regional tier would be in their best interests and reduce the need for allegedly inexperienced (in health matters) civil servants to engage in management functions *vis-à-vis* the NHS, in England there is a growing body of opinion that questions the need for RHAs as presently constituted. Indeed, as mentioned, the Government may review the regional function once the present changes have been completed. There is general consensus that regional functions exist in England but that RHAs may not be the most appropriate instrument for dispensing them. One possibility, floated in *Patients First*,[56] is that, in future, regional bodies might be composed of DHA representatives. There is concern that if RHAs continue unchanged now that the smaller DHAs have been established then it is possible that the Government's aim of greater local discretion and automomy will be thwarted as functions, which some authorities will find it difficult to run, are sucked up to region. More generally, there is evidence to suggest that RHAs, in their present form, remain detached from local services as well as uncertain of their role.[57]

Since the first reorganisation of the NHS in the 1970s, the district tier has performed differently in the four countries. In England, former District Management Teams (DMTs) were directly accountable to AHAs and not to the Area Team of Officers (ATOs), whereas elsewhere in the UK district teams (or groups) are accountable to area teams (or groups) and not directly to the area authorities (or boards). Further, in Scotland, the emergence of the structure below area level was greatly influenced by area boards. Not only do health boards in Scotland have more direct authority over districts (as was previously the case in Wales and Northern Ireland), but the areas played a major role in defining and restructuring the districts in the first place. In England, area officers *monitored* their district counterparts, who were accountable to AHAs, but this relationship was not a managerial (i.e. superior–subordinate) one. Elsewhere in the UK, the relationship was (and still is in Scotland) strictly hierarchical. Districts in England, therefore, had a totally different status from districts elsewhere in the UK. This is evident in the greater independence they enjoyed and in their planning role. These factors may account, in part, for the decision to establish DHAs in England, which, in most places, have been substituted for DMTs, and to create more single-district areas in other parts of the UK where districts were never of the same status. While districts in England should gain from the latest reforms, their relationship with RHAs, as mentioned above, will determine how far they are able to operate independently.

There are important differences between the four countries in the composition of management teams. Area Executive Teams (AETs) in Northern Ireland show the greatest differences, in part reflecting the integrated structure between health and PSS operating there. As elsewhere in the UK, the teams in Northern Ireland operate as consensus-forming bodies. Until recently, there were four members with executive authority – an administrator, a medical officer, a nursing officer and a director of social services – and a fifth member representing the interests of hospital consultants and GPs. As one of the latest reforms, a sixth member of the team is to be added so that there will be separate representation for hospital consultants and GPs. Teams elsewhere in the UK have four members. A second key difference in Northern Ireland is that the administrative officer is also the accounting officer. This tradition is similar to the joint post of Secretary and Treasurer which was a notable feature of the Scottish Health Service before 1974. The post no longer survives in Scotland and there are those[58] who believe that finance officers should become full members of the executive team in Northern Ireland. A final key difference between management teams in the four services concerns the form, and strength, of medical representation on teams. In the case of Northern Ireland, as noted, this is being strengthened.

Until 1982, the operation of management teams (or groups) varied between the four countries. Some of these differences remain a feature of the new structure; others have disappeared, perhaps to be replaced by new ones. It is not possible to predict what may happen, particularly at unit level. Certainly guidance from the health departments has varied in its degree of specificity between the four countries. For example, in Scotland, the Secretary of State has left health boards to devise appropriate unit structures with a minimum of guidance. He only requires to be informed of boards' plans. This *laissez-faire* approach is in marked contrast to what has happened in Wales and Northern Ireland. The Welsh Office has asked health authorities to submit their plans for units for scrutiny and approval. In addition, detailed guidance on the principles of management at district and unit levels was issued in late 1981 by the Welsh Office to the new health authorities. A similar interventionist approach has been adopted in Northern Ireland, with the DHSS (NI) keeping a close watch over the NHS. Practice in England resembles that in Scotland, with regions supervising developments in place of health boards.

Differences exist in the management of the NHS in the four constituent parts of the UK. As the new structure settles down it is possible that other differences will emerge. Whether these differences relate to the organisation, composition or operation of health authorities, they may well have implications for member–officer relations, for policy formulation and implementation, for relations between different levels and so on. Detailed examination of the variations to assess whether or not they have an impact on priorities and service provision in the separate countries may be useful since, as mentioned, no work of this kind exists on an intra-UK basis.

Planning

The tripartite structure for health services in the UK which survived from 1948 to 1974 was no planner's dream. Reorganisation of the NHS, which occurred at a time when a planning mood had manifested itself in various parts of the public sector, was intended to encourage, and facilitate, planning both in order to achieve a better use of resources and to ensure that priorities long advocated by successive governments were attained. The tendency on the part of those charged with reorganising the NHS, especially in England, was to favour a planning approach related to rational models of policy-making that were fashionable at the time. There was a desire to move beyond 'disjointed incrementalism' and 'muddling through' and a belief, again held most strongly in England, that the centre's ability to control the distribution of resources needed to be strengthened in order that priority groups in the 'Cinderella' sectors (i.e. the elderly, the mentally ill, the mentally handicapped, children) would receive resources that had been denied them over the years by allegedly powerful field health authorities under the control of acute medical specialities.[59]

Although health services (and PSS) planning has been a dominant theme in all four countries since 1974, it has been pursued in England with a zeal not evident to the same extent in the rest of the UK. Like management, planning has a slightly different meaning, or emphasis, depending on where you happen to be. The machinery also differs between countries in the UK, reflecting these rather different approaches.

The planning system in England has now been modified following criticism of previous arrangements[60] and to fall in line with the Governments commitment to enhance local discretion. *Patients First*[61] referred to the then existing planning arrangements as being 'over-complicated and bureaucratic'. However critics of the simplified arrangements[62] do not believe they tackle the real issues which underlay the shortcomings of the planning system that was originally introduced in 1976. Planning arrangements elsewhere in the UK have not been disturbed.

In Wales and Northern Ireland, broadly similar approaches to planning exist. The respective planning systems cannot be described here in detail. It is sufficient to note that, apart from different time-scales, both countries share a commitment to comprehensive planning, to programmes of care, to the issuance of central guidelines and to the preparation of strategic and operational plans by health authorities. In Northern Ireland, of course, the planning system covers PSS at the sub-national level as well as at national level. On balance, there is little substantively different about the planning systems between England, Wales and Northern Ireland. Nevertheless, there is scope for research which seeks to explore the variations that do exist. It may be that there are greater differences than appear from a perusal of the relevant literature. Moreover, the planning systems in each of the countries operate within a different set of structural and interpersonal arrangements.

In the 1982 reorganisation, the Welsh Office speculated in its consultation document[64] on the suggestion that an advisory Welsh Health Council be set up. It was claimed that such a body would obviate the need for a regional health authority for Wales. The Council would represent all health authorities, advise the Secretary of State and take a lead role in strategic planning. This proposal was rejected and instead a series of formal meetings between the Minister, AHA chairmen and representatives of other interests is to be introduced along the lines of the multi-board forum in Northern Ireland. Had a Health Council been established, it would have resembled the Scottish Health Service Planning Council described below.

In Scotland, planning for health does seem to have taken a different direction. Certainly, in thinking about planning, and in some of the apparatus created, this would appear to be so. Whereas planning for health in the other three countries is intended to be *comprehensive*, in Scotland *strategic* planning has been emphasised[65] which is suggestive of a more flexible, selective approach. The Scottish Institute for Operational Research (SIOR), now defunct, worked closely with the SHHD on the development of planning processes for the NHS and devised a scheme based on Etzioni's 'mixed-scanning' approach.[66] This approach deliberately sets out to avoid the comprehensive ideal of the rationalists by recognising the inevitable constraints present in any decision-making environment. The approach favoured by the SIOR comprises three key elements: (i) a periodic review process to identify major issues; (ii) a selection process to identify important issues that justify detailed planning attention; and (iii) a participative approach which involves all interested parties. From this skeletal outline, it would appear that the planning approach that is being developed in Scotland does not possess the centralising tendencies, or technocratic rigour (at any rate in theory), of the English system. Some evidence for this can be gleaned from the various priorities documents produced by the four central departments between 1976 and 1977.[67] Of these, only the two English ones, in particular the first, specified in detail through the setting of targets by how much the priority services were expected to grow. The other documents in the other countries dealt only with broad principles.

However, the priorities document issued in 1981 by the DHSS is notable for its lack of specificity and for a *laissez-faire* approach to planning. Ironically, it has much in common with the other priorities documents produced in the mid-1970s in the rest of the UK. *Care in Action* does not set definite targets for developments in services and its whole emphasis is on adapting national priorities to local circumstances. In contrast, the SHHD published *Scottish Health Authorities Priorities for the Eighties* in 1980 which is more than twice the length of its English counterpart and an altogether more substantial document. In broad terms, the approach is akin to that adopted for the English priorities documents of the mid-1970s. The document, prepared by the Scottish Health Service Planning Council, and possibly its first major piece of work, is comprehensive and thorough. A programme budgeting approach is used (no longer a feature of the English document) and different priority areas are suggested depending on whether there is a 0, 1.5 or 3% growth rate in the next few years. This is an interesting attempt to retain flexibility in planning and to acknowledge uncertainty by generating a range of alternative scenarios.

As Mooney has remarked: 'It seems therefore that, while DHSS is giving the regions greater leeway than in the past in deciding the extent to which they pursue national priorities, the Scottish Department is tending in the opposite direction.'[68] Mooney also notes the emphasis in the English document on efficiency in resource use and on the role of private medicine. The Scottish document refers fleetingly to one but makes no mention of the other.

Reorganisation of the Scottish Health Service in 1974 saw the creation of a new agency in the central administration of the health service, the Scottish Health Service Planning Council (SHSPC). It has no identical counterpart elsewhere in the UK. The SHSPC comprises representatives from health boards, universities and the SHHD and is designed to involve health boards directly in national policy-making. The Council advises the Secretary of State on planning matters and does so through national consultative committees of the health care professions and through its own multi-disciplinary programme planning groups. Within the SHHD itself, a health service planning unit has been set up which, together with the Planning Council Secretariat, constitutes the Planning Group. The purpose of these elaborate arrangements is to ensure that while there is strong central involvement in planning, the way the Planning Council and other machinery have been constituted is a guarantee against health planning becoming over-centralised. In an unpublished memorandum written to the Royal Commission on the NHS, the Chairman of the Planning Council observes that 'since there is no readily available comprehensive and quantified package for setting priorities, it would seem that there is no alternative to having inputs from a range of perspectives and viewpoints'. He also suggests that the Planning Council 'is a bridging mechanism, or intermediate structure, between the central and local aspects of the health service . . .'[69]

In the UK, little is known about planning for health at the sub-national level. Programme planning groups, or their equivalent, have been established by health authorities in the four countries. These are multidisciplinary and are concerned with particular client groups, normally the elderly, mentally ill and children. The programme planning groups at area level in Scotland and Northern Ireland mirror those operating nationally. In England, Joint Care Planning Teams at area level fulfilled a similar purpose and there were, in addition, District Planning Teams denoting the importance of this level. What will happen in the new structure remains to be seen. Arrangements have yet to be worked out. Although the DHSS in England recommended that a programme budgeting (PB) approach be adopted at local level, not many areas in England appear to have achieved much in this direction.[70] Some progress has, however, been made in Scotland, where a PB system developed at Aberdeen is being applied in other health boards with the SHHD's support.

The nature of health planning, which has only been skated over in this section, offers many opportunities for comparative research. An obvious area to probe is the extent to which Scottish practice is different from the rest of the UK and, if there are marked differences, why this should be so. If it is a matter of size, i.e. because Scotland is of manageable proportions it can afford to adopt a more flexible stance, then surely Wales and Northern Ireland are in a similar position. Yet they have both taken a lead from England which, in the case of Northern Ireland, is particularly interesting for it usually looks to Scotland. A second issue concerns the changing views of planning and priorities which, as has been mentioned, is especially marked between England and Scotland since the publication of their most recent priorities documents. It is by no means clear why this shift in philosophy has occurred or whether it is a significant development or not. Now that norms are being used in Scotland for planning purposes, they may have implications for health boards and their relations with the centre. Glennerster, writing about the English priorities documents of the mid-1970s, expressed concern over the domination of planning by bed-population norms and staffing ratios and over the thrust of plans to achieve congruence with national norms. 'If we had some efficiency criterion for adopting these norms in the first place the process might be less worrying though even that is doubtful, given the variations in conditions that apply.'[71] Glennerster's main concern is that planning might rigidify the development of health services, and render them less responsive. It will be interesting to see if Scotland can manage to avoid these potential pitfalls. Moreover, there may be implications here for the different planning systems operating in the UK.

Comment and conclusions

The fact that differences between the four health services, and hence the four countries, in the UK may not appear so distinctive when the pattern of relationships is compared with inter-governmental relations in, say, countries with a federal system of government, does not mean that the differences that do exist are unimportant. It may be that research of a 'middle range' variety is less glamorous than elaborate, macro trans-national projects but it is certainly no less relevant. Glennerster believes that the penchant among academics for 'macrotheorising' may have led to a neglect of more 'traditional questions', including:

> how is the service working, who is it reaching, who is it not reaching, what are the consequences of delivering the service in one way compared to another, what differences do alternative administrative structures make, . . . what are the obstacles to access, what are the resource constraints and what criteria can be used to debate priorities?[72]

In similar vein, Kogan has argued that policy analysts are preoccupied

> with the largest animals in the political science zoo. Money is spent, decisions are made, professionals exert power, clientele receive services (or do not receive them) in a vast web of institutions. It is high time that . . . analysts stopped worrying about the Think Tank, or Cabinet, or the Treasury and started to look at the sites of the real social action.[73]

An examination of the different health care delivery systems operating in the UK would go some way towards meeting Glennerster's and Kogan's criticisms.

Mapping administrative permutations can be no more than a small first step in the task of investigating their implications for health policy delivery. The NHS may *look* different in the constituent parts of the UK but *is* it different in practice? Identifying the differences does not, by itself, provide an answer to the 'so what?' variety of question, although it is a useful educational device for dispelling ignorance about the NHS in the UK. For example, there is evidence to support the view that the resource allocation formulae in use in England to redress regional imbalances have been, and are being, subverted by local health authorities and the machinations of local decision actors.[74] But to what extent, if any, do differences in structure contribute to this finding? It might be postulated that such distortions are more likely to occur in the English Service with its lengthy chain of command stretching from the centre to the periphery. Such a cumbersome arrangement may render local decision processes less visible to scrutiny by higher levels. In Wales, Scotland and Northern Ireland, the opportunities to subvert their respective resource allocation formulae may not be so readily available because what happens locally may be more visible to higher management levels, given the absence of a regional tier.

Reference has been made to the complex pattern of relationships that prevails within and between the four health services in the UK. If anything, the true situation is understated. Yet these 'issue networks',[75] which are a feature of all public policy-making, are a crucial factor in the NHS's evolution. They are in need of unravelling if the true dynamics of the policy process, whether in health or in other areas, are to be fully comprehended. The 'professional–bureaucratic complex' in health care is undergoing continuous mutation: witness the growth of skills and specialisms making for fragmentation and problems of coordination. This complex comprises many elements, the key ones being: (i) relationships between central agencies; (ii) relationships between local agencies; (iii) relationships between central and local agencies; and (iv) relationships between service providers and clients. In the interstices of these relationships are located numerous bodies some of which may be found only in one country, while others may have equivalents in other countries comprising the UK. In addition to official bodies such as, for instance, the Health Advisory Service[76] and the Health Education Council are interest groups such as Age Concern, MIND and the Child Poverty Action Group as well as locally based voluntary groups. Then there are the media – newspapers, professional journals and broadcasters – at national and local levels. One way of studying the operation of these 'policy networks', and their implications for democratic politics and public accountability, would be to look at them on a comparative basis within the UK. Such a breakdown would render the task more manageable and provide an opportunity to observe their operations in a variety of settings.

Underlying most of the points made in this chapter have been two principal themes: (i) the nature of central–local relations in the NHS, both within each country and between the 'centre' (i.e. the Whitehall/Westminster axis) in London and the centres in other countries; and (ii) the nature of policy formation and implementation in the NHS and the effect of the different intra-UK administrative arrangements and professional practices on service provision and patient care.

The full extent, and nature, of the various differences between the four health services operating in the UK have not been conveyed here, nor could they be in the space available. Hopefully, the selection of themes and issues has been sufficient to show that there are many differences, mainly of a middle-range type, between the four countries, some of which may, in fact, be quite fundamental reflecting, as they do, differing traditions, problems and settings. Some of these differences, like the growth of the private health sector in parts of England, could become more significant in future.

It has been suggested that comparative research might usefully proceed along three dimensions: structure, process and output. The focus of this chapter has been on structure and process factors although the full extent of similarities and differences within each of these categories remains to be explored, particularly from an organisational and political perspective. This chapter has indicated areas where comparative research from such a perspective might be productive, although the list is by no means exhaustive. There are various ways in which health care systems in the UK might be studied comparatively. Groups of patients, particularly in geriatrics and psychiatry, are the responsibility of many different agencies. New delivery forms to meet problems have resulted in day hospitals, halfway houses, assessment and special rehabilitation units and so on. It is not clear how all these forms of care work together under a range of differing circumstances and professional ideologies within the four health care systems operating in the UK. It may be that 'the organisational differences are more a matter of form than of substance and exert little influence on the way decisions are actually made',[77] although this in itself would be an interesting finding given the propensity among policy-makers for constant institutional rejigging of the kind that has been, is being, and doubtless will be, witnessed.

In looking specifically at the problems of intra and inter-agency collaboration between countries, a 'bottom-up' approach might be appropriate; that is, one which takes as its starting point a client group and uses it as a 'tracer' through the social care system in order to penetrate the 'black box', in which inputs are translated into outputs, and to unravel the system of administrative politics within. An example of a study (but not a comparative one) which begins to approach these matters is Blaxter's investigation of the needs of the disabled in which she discusses the importance of inter-agency relationships.[78] Alternatively, budgetary processes provide a means of studying how agencies in the health field allocate resources and set priorities and the importance, or otherwise, of different organisational settings.

There remains considerable ignorance over the efficacy of particular organisational arrangements in the NHS, partly because their dynamics are insufficiently understood. Yet, within the UK, there exist unexplained and unexplored variations. Indeed, these may become more significant in future, for it appears that current developments in England mark a shift away from the ideal of an integrated health service, a major theme of the 1974 NHS reorganisation, while the other countries making up the UK remain wedded to this ideal. Also, in regard to planning there are the beginnings of potentially significant differences. The *laissez-faire* approach being adopted in England is not being echoed elsewhere. Clearly, the study of health services within the UK could prove fruitful.

Notes

1. See, for example, E. Jaques (ed.), *Health Services*, London: Heinemann, 1978; W. J. M. Mackenzie, *Power and Responsibility in Health Care*, Oxford: Oxford University Press, 1979; and R. Klein, 'Costs and Benefits of Complexity: The British National Health Service', in R. Rose (ed.), *Challenge to Governance: Studies in Overloaded Polities*, London: Sage, 1980.
2. See, for example, the Nuffield Centre for Health Services Studies' evaluation (*Towards a New Rationality: A Study of Planning in the NHS*, Vols. 1–4, Leeds: University of Leeds, 1979) of the NHS planning system in two regions in England. Similar work has been completed at the Institute for Health Studies: see, *inter alia*, H. Elcock and Stuart Haywood, *The Buck Stops Where? Accountability and Control in the National Health Service*, Hull: University of Hull, 1980; and S. Haywood and A. Alaszewski, *Crisis in the Health Service*, London: Croom Helm, 1980.
3. R. Taylor, 'The local health system: an ethnography of interest groups and decision-making', *Social Science and Medicine*, Vol. II, 1977, and 'The local health system: observations on the exercise of professional influence', *Health and Social Service Journal*, Centre Eight Papers, 21 July 1978; C. Wiseman, 'Selection of Major Planning Issues', *Policy Sciences*, Vol. 9, 1978, and 'Policy Making in the Scottish Health Services at National Level', in N. Drucker and H. M. Drucker (eds.), *The Scottish Government Yearbook 1980*, Edinburgh: Paul Harris, 1979, and 'Strategic Planning in the Scottish Health Service – A Mixed-Scanning Approach', *Long Range Planning*, Vol. 12, April 1979; and David J. Hunter, 'Coping with uncertainty: decisions and resources within health authorities', *Sociology of Health and Illness*, Vol. 1, June 1979; 'Practice: decisions and resources in the National Health Service (Scotland)', in K. M. Boyd (ed.), *The Ethics of Resource Allocation in Health Care*, Edinburgh: University of Edinburgh Press, 1979; Policy-making in Area Health Boards: The Role of the Board Member', in H. M. Drucker and N. L. Drucker (eds.), *The Scottish Government Yearbook 1981*, Edinburgh: Paul Harris,

1980; and *Coping with Uncertainty: Policy and Politics in the National Health Service*, Chichester: Research Studies Press, Wiley, 1980.
4. R. Rose, *Northern Ireland: A Time of Choice*, London: Macmillan, 1976, p.15.
5. See B. Rodgers with A. Doran and M. Jones, *The Study of Social Policy: A Comparative Approach*, London: Allen and Unwin, 1979.
6. H. M. Leichter, *A Comparative Approach to Policy Analysis: Health Care Policy in Four Nations*, Cambridge: Cambridge University Press, 1979.
7. See also A. J. Heidenheimer *et al.*, *Comparative Public Policy*, London: Macmillan, 1976.
8. D. Owen, 'Reflections on the Royal Commission', The Trevor Lloyd Hughes Memorial Lecture, 25 October 1979, unpublished.
9. Royal Commission on the National Health Service, *Report*, Cmnd 7615, London: HMSO, 1979, p. 15.
10. *Report*, p. 214.
11. Ibid.
12. *Report*, p. 26.
13. *Report*, p. 14.
14. Sir George Godber, 'Regional Devolution and the NHS', in E. Craven (ed.), *Regional Devolutoin and Social Policy*, London: Centre for Studies in Social Policy, Macmillan, 1975, p. 72.
15. Godber, p. 84.
16. J. G. Kellas, *The Scottish Political System*, 2nd edn., London: Cambridge University Press, 1975; A. Maynard and A. Ludbrook, 'Budget Allocation in the National Health Service', *Journal of Social Policy*, Vol. 9, no. 3, 1980, and 'What's Wrong with the National Health Service?', *Lloyds Bank Review*, no. 138, October 1980.
17. Department of Health and Social Security, *Sharing Resources for Health in England*, report of the Resource Allocation Working Party (RAWP), London: HMSO, 1976.
18. Welsh Office, *Report of the Steering Committee on Resource Allocation in Wales*, Cardiff: HMSO, 1977; Scottish Home and Health Department, *Scottish Health Authorities Revenue Equalisation*, Report of the Working Party on Revenue Resource Allocation, Edinburgh: HMSO, 1977; and DHSS (NI), *Proposals for the Allocation of Revenue Resources for Health and Personal Social Services*, report of the working group on revenue resource allocations to health and social services boards in Northern Ireland, Belfast: HMSO, 1978.
19. Maynard and Ludbrook, 'What's Wrong with the National Health Service?', p. 40.
20. Maynard and Ludbrook, 'What's Wrong with the National Health Service?', p. 39.
21. A. Maynard and A. Ludbrook, 'Budget Allocation in the National Health Service', unpublished paper presented at conference on health care expenditure, Milan, October 1981, pp. 21–5.
22. *Report*, p. 145.
23. M. Lipsky, 'Standing the Study of Public Policy Implementation on its Head', in W. D. Burnham and M. W. Weinberg (eds.), *American Politics and Public Policy*, Cambridge, Mass.: MIT Press, 1978; Social Science Research Council, *Central–Local Government Relationships*, a panel report to the Research Initiatives Board, London: 1979.
24. Politics of Health Group, *Going Private*, London: 1981.
25 P. R. Torrens, 'Health Insurance in the United States: Implications for the United Kingdom', *The Lancet*, 5 January 1980; B. Abel-Smith, 'Towards a healthier population', *New Society*, 15 October 1981.
26. *Report*, p. 294.
27. R. Klein, 'Health Services', in P. M. Jackson (ed.), *Government Policy Initiatives 1979–80: Some Case Studies in Public Administration*, London: RIPA, 1981.
28. DHSS and Welsh Office, *Patients First*, London: HMSO, 1979.

29. SHHD, *Structure and Management of the NHS in Scotland*, Edinburgh: HMSO, 1979.
30. DHSS (NI), *Consultative Paper on the Structure and Management of Health and Personal Social Services in Northern Ireland*, Belfast: HMSO, 1979.
31. DHSS, Circular HC (80)8, 1980.
32. SHHD, Circular 1981 (GEN)14.
33. Welsh Office, *The Structure and Management of the NHS in Wales*, Cardiff: HMSO, 1980; DHSS (NI), *Report of the Advisory Group on the Structure and Management of Health and Personal Social Services in Northern Ireland*, Belfast: February 1981.
34. Welsh Office, Circular WHC (81)8, 1981.
35. DHSS (NI), Circular HSS(P) 1/81, 1981.
36. A. G. Davis, 'An Unequivocal Change of Policy: Prevention, Health and Medical Sociology', *Social Science and Medicine*, Vol. 13A, March 1979.
37. Report of the Committee on Local Authority and Allied Personal Social Services (Chairman: Lord Seebohm), London: HMSO, 1968.
38. SHHD, *Reorganisation of the Scottish Health Service*, Cmnd 4734, London: HMSO, 1971, p. 14.
39. SHHD, *Report*, Working Party on Relationships between Health Boards and Local Authorities, Edinburgh: HMSO, 1977.
40. G. Wistow and A. Webb, *Patients First: One Step Backwards for Collaboration?*, Loughborough: Loughborough University, 1980.
41. DHSS, *Care in the Community: A consultative document on Moving Resources for Care in England*, London: HMSO, 1981.
42. DHSS (NI), *Strategy for the Development of Health and Personal Social Services in Northern Ireland*, Belfast: HMSO, 1975; DHSS, *Priorities for Health and Personal Social Services in England – A Consultative Document*, London: HMSO, 1976; Welsh Office, *Proposed All Wales Policies and Priorities for the Planning and Provision of Health and Personal Social Services from 1976/77 to 1979/80, A Consultative Document*, Cardiff: 1976; DHSS, *Priorities in the Health and Social Services: The Way Forward*, London, HMSO, 1977, and *Care in Action: A Handbook of Policies and Priorities for the Health and Personal Social Services in England*, London: HMSO, 1981.
43. SHHD, *The Health Service in Scotland: The Way Ahead*, Edinburgh: HMSO, 1976, and *Scottish Health Authorities' Priorities for the Eighties*, Edinburgh: HMSO, 1980.
44. Wiseman, 'Policy Making in the Scottish Health Services at National Level', p. 145.
45. Circular HSS(P) 1/81, para 11, p. 4.
46. *Report*, p. 327.
47. M. Kogan *et al.*, *The Working of the National Health Service*, The Royal Commission on the NHS, Research Paper Number 1, London: HMSO, 1978, p. 69.
48. K. Newton, 'Is Small Really So Beautiful? Is Big Really So Ugly?', *Studies in Public Policy No 18*, Centre for the Study of Public Policy, Glasgow: University of Strathclyde, 1978.
49. R. Klein, 'Policy-Making in the National Health Service', *Political Studies*, Vol. 22, no. 1, 1974.
50. DHSS, *Management Arrangements for the Reorganised National Health Service*, London: HMSO, 1972; Welsh Office, *Management Arrangements for the Reorganised National Health Service in Wales*, Cardiff: HMSO, 1972; Booz, Allen and Hamilton, *An Integrated Service: The Reorganisation of Health and Personal Social Services in Northern Ireland*, February 1972.
51. SHHD, *Administrative Practice of Hospital Boards in Scotland* (Farquharson–Lang Report), Edinburgh: HMSO, 1966.
52. K. Barnard, 'Health planning – the last of the panaceas', in K. Barnard and K. Lee (eds.), *NHS Reorganisation: Issues and Prospects*, Leeds: University of Leeds, 1974.
53. Welsh Office, *The Structure and Management of the NHS in Wales*.

54. DHSS (NI), *Consultative Paper on the Structure and Management of Health and Personal Social Services in Northern Ireland*. As a concession the DHSS (NI) has set up a multi-board consultative forum to act as 'an informal clearing-house for the exchange and coordination of views' (circular HSS(P) 1/81, para 31, p. 9). It has no executive functions or authority.
55. SHHD, *Structure and Management of the NHS in Scotland*.
56. DHSS and Welsh Office, 1979.
57. H. Elcock, 'Regional Government in Action: The Members of Two Regional Health Authorities', *Public Administration*, Vol. 56, Winter 1978.
58. J. Perrin *et al*., *Management of Financial Resources in the National Health Service*, The Royal Commission on the NHS, Research Paper Number 2, London: HMSO, 1978.
59. R. H. S. Crossman, *A Politician's View of Health Service Planning*, Glasgow: University of Glasgow, 1972.
60. K. Barnard *et al*., 'NHS planning: as assessment', *Hospital and Health Services Review*, Vol. 76, August and September 1980.
61. DHSS and Welsh Office, 1979.
62. For example, D. Irving *et al*., 'Planning Inaction', *Hospital and Health Services Review*, Vol. 77, April 1981.
63. Welsh Office, *Health Service Planning: A Short Guide*, Cardiff: HMSO, 1975; DHSS (NI), *Strategy for the Development of Health and Personal Social Services in Northern Ireland*; Circular HSS(P) 1/81. The planning system in Northern Ireland commenced in 1982.
64. *The Structure and Management of the NHS in Wales*.
65. Wiseman, 'Strategic Planning in the Scottish Health Service – A Mixed-Scanning Approach'.
66. Wiseman, 'Selection of Major Planning Issues', 'Policy Making in the Scottish Health Services at National Level', and 'Strategic Planning in the Scottish Health Service – A Mixed-Scanning Approach'.
67. DHSS (NI), *Strategy for the Development of Health and Personal Social Services in Northern Ireland*, Belfast: HMSO; DHSS, *Priorities for Health and Personal Social Services: The Way Forward*; Welsh Office, *Proposed All Wales Policies and Priorities for the Planning and Provision of Health and Personal Social Services from 1976/77 to 1979/80, A Consultative Document*; and SHHD, *The Health Service in Scotland: The Way Ahead*.
68. G. Mooney, 'Efficient Care', *Public Money*, June 1981, pp. 7–8.
69. See K. Lee and A. Mills, 'The contribution of economics to health service planning', *Health and Social Service Journal*, Centre Eight Papers, 8 February 1979.
70. Scottish Health Service Planning Council, *The Role of the Scottish Health Service Planning Council*, memorandum to the Royal Commission on the NHS, unpublished, 1979. The same point is made by T. D. Hunter, 'Planning for Health – the role of the Scottish Health Service Planning Council', *Hospital and Health Services Review*, Vol. 75, May 1974, pp. 168–71.
71. H. Glennerster, 'The Development of Social Planning in the United Kingdom', unpublished paper prepared for SSRC Workshop on Policy, Planning and Implementation in Social Policy, School for Advanced Urban Studies, Bristol, March 1979, p. 12.
72. H. Glennerster, *Social Service Budgets and Social Policy*, London: Allen & Unwin, 1975.
73. M. Kogan, 'Notes and Comments', *British Journal of Political Science*, Vol. 6, 1976, p. 508.
74. Elcock and Haywood, *The Buck Stops Where?*
75. H. Heclo, 'Issue Networks and the Executive Establishment', in A. King (ed.), *The New American Political System*, Washington: American Enterprise Institute, 1978, and A. G. Jordan, 'Iron Triangles, Woolly Corporatism and Elastic

Nets: Images of the Policy Process', *Journal of Public Policy*, Vol. 1, 1981.

76. This body covers England and Wales; it monitors preformance in the long stay care sector (i.e. the elderly and the mentally ill). Scotland has its own Hospital Advisory Service which, as the title suggests, excludes community care services. Northern Ireland is contemplating whether to establish a similar body.
77. Perrin *et al.*, *Management of Financial Resources in the National Health Service*.
78. M. Blaxter, *The Meaning of Disability*, London: Heinemann, 1976.

6 The Allocation of Health Care Resources in the United Kingdom

Alan Maynard and *Anne Ludbrook*

Introduction

An unequal regional distribution of resources in the National Health Service (NHS) was inherited in 1948, when the voluntary (non-profit) organisations and local government handed over to the state the control of a hospital system which was characterised by an uneven distribution in the quality and quantity of the bed stock. During the early years of the NHS, the resources that were available were divided amongst the Regional Hospital Boards (RHB) broadly in proportion to their expenditure in the last year for which figures were available and this *ad hoc* incremental procedure tended to maintain the existing inequalities.

In the 1960s, the first attempt was made to reduce the geographical inequalities in the distribution of hospital beds. The capital building programme[1] was ambitious but progress was slow because of the limited funds available. The next plan to achieve a better distribution of resources was formulated in the late 1960s and involved the redistribution of revenue rather than capital. The hospital revenue allocation formula was introduced in 1970 in England and formed the basis of regional allocations from 1971 until it was superseded by the proposals of the Resource Allocation Working Party interim report.[2] The full report appeared the following year and similar reports have subsequently been published for the other constituent nations of the UK. These reports are the result of the establishment of various working parties with the specific objective of devising methods of resource allocation that would ensure equal access to services for those in equal need. The working parties interpreted this objective as the equalisation of financial capacity to provide services for those in equal need.

The purpose of this paper is to analyse critically the development and implementation of these new resource allocation systems in the health systems of England, Scotland, Wales and Northern Ireland. This paper is divided into four sections. The first section sets out the elements of the formulae used to allocate resources in England, Scotland, Wales and Northern Ireland: the English Resource Allocation Working Party formula

(RAWP), the Scottish Health Authorities Revenue Equalisation formula (SHARE), the Steering Committee on Resource Allocations in Wales (SCRAW) and the Northern Ireland Proposals for the Allocation of Revenue Resources formula (PARR). The second section examines the criticisms that have been made of these formulae and reviews the effects of their implementation. The next section reviews the policy issues that remain and the final section summarises the chapter and offers some conclusions.

The formula approach to resource allocation – the proposals

In this section our objective is to provide a brief outline of the proposals for resource allocation presented in the four reports, RAWP,[3] SHARE,[4] SCRAW[5] and PARR[6]. All four reports adopt the same broad principle that resource allocations should be based on population size, weighted to reflect the need for services. They differ, to some extent, in their methods of weighting the populations and in the services included in the formula allocations. The proposals for each service area will be considered in turn, starting with those that feature in all four reports.

The elements of the formulae

(*1*) *Non-psychiatric in-patient services* The RAWP report proposes that Regional Health Authority (RHA) populations should be weighted by national bed utilisation rates for each age group, sex and condition. As a proxy for relative morbidity, these are adjusted by the standardised fertility ratio (SFR) for conditions of pregnancy (ICD, Chapter XI), and by the condition specific standardised mortality ratio (SMR) for all other non-psychiatric conditions except skin diseases (ICD, Chapter XII). The SCRAW report weights area populations by the average annual cost of non-psychiatric in-patient care for each age/sex group and by the overall SMR.

SHARE and PARR treat non-obstetric and obstetric services separately. For the former, the weighting factors differ from those in RAWP in that the overall SMRs are used; the use of condition specific SMRs is felt to be inappropriate in Scotland, Wales and Northern Ireland because of the smaller number of deaths involved. In addition, the SHARE report recommends that SMRs be applied only to the population aged under 65, arguing that morbidity and mortality are more closely associated in younger age groups. For obstetric services, SHARE and PARR recommend sharing the total population between the Health Boards in proportion to expected use, determined by the number of births in each maternal age group weighted by the national bed use per birth for each age group.

(2) *Day and out-patient services* The basic weighting factors used in all the reports are the utilisation of services by age and sex and the overall SMR. The RAWP report recommends that the SMR be applied to non-psychiatric patients only and the SHARE report restricts its use to those aged under 65.

(3) *Community health services* The four reports recommend that population should be weighted for utilisation by age, adjusted by the overall SMR. SHARE applies SMRs only to those aged under 65 and both SHARE and PARR apply a sparsity factor to certain community services.

(4) *In-patient services for the mentally ill and mentally handicapped* RAWP, SHARE and PARR weight the populations for bed utilisation by age, sex and, for mental illness only, marital status. These services are excluded from the SCRAW formula.

(5) *Ambulance services* These are included in the RAWP, SCRAW and PARR formulas. All three reports recommend using overall SMRs to weight populations but SCRAW and PARR also use sparsity factors; road miles per head of population in Wales and the ratio of local to national average miles per patient carried in Northern Ireland.

(6) *Family Practitioner Committee (FPC) administration* This is included only in the RAWP formula, and the allocation is based on unadjusted population.

(7) *Personal social services* These are included in the PARR formula only. Allocations for services for the handicapped are made in proportion to the number of mentally and physically handicapped persons in each Board. The allocations for services for the elderly and for general services take account of indicators of need from the 1971 Census and sparsity factors.

(8) *Combining the weighted populations* The basic revenue allocation is determined by combining the various weighted populations in proportion to recent revenue expenditure on each service. The final allocations are arrived at after adjustments have been made for cross-boundary flows, for teaching costs and, in the case of Scotland and Northern Ireland, minor adjustments for other special services (mainly laboratory services).

(*9*) *Cross boundary flows* The RAWP and SCRAW reports allow for in-patient flows between regions, costed on a national specialty basis. For day and out-patients, only formal agency relationships are taken into account in the RAWP formula. The SCRAW formula allows for out-patient flows, on the basis of a sample survey. SHARE and PARR both recommend that in-patient flows should be costed at the average cost for the group of hospitals in which the receiving hospital is classified, except that in the case of teaching hospitals the average cost for an equivalent non-teaching group should be used. The adjustment for day and out-patients assumes that the cross-boundary flow is proportional to that for in-patients.

(*10*) *Teaching costs* The allowance in the RAWP formula to cover the excess clinical costs of teaching, the Service Increment for Teaching (SIFT), is taken to be 75% of the median excess cost of teaching hospitals.[7] The SIFT is distributed in proportion to student numbers. In Wales, the teaching allowance is based on the difference in costs between provincial teaching hospitals and other large acute hospitals in England and Wales. Actual costs of supra-area services are allowed for separately.

In Scotland and Northern Ireland, the total excess cost of teaching centres is allocated separately. SHARE recommends that the Additional Costs of Teaching (ACT) should be assumed to be the same for each undergraduate in Scotland as in England and that the total teaching allowance should be allocated according to student numbers. The remaining excess cost of teaching centres (approximately 40%) is allocated according to the size of the composite weighted population served by each teaching centre. Additional adjustments are made for supra-area services provided by non-teaching hospitals. The PARR report adopts the same approach, in principle, but as all teaching and regional services are concentrated under one Board, the distinction between teaching and non-teaching services is not necessary.

(*11*) *Capital allocations* Of the four reports reviewed here, only RAWP has tackled capital redistribution using the same basic framework as for revenue. Target allocations are based on the weighted populations (1)–(5) above, except that for community services the age weights are replaced by GP consultation rates by age and sex. The base population is projected five years ahead and the populations are combined in proportion to the expected expenditure on each service over the following three years. Some cross-boundary flows are taken into account by cross-accounting between regions but in general they are ignored as they are, in part, attributable to a lack of facilities in the exporting region. The total estimated capital stock of the NHS, expressed in terms of the 1975 replacement cost, is notionally distributed between the RHAs in accordance with their weighted population share to produce target capital stock allocations. The RAWP report recommends that up to 1986/87 amounts varying between 10 and 30% of the total capital budget should be allocated between regions with an historic capital stock deficit. The remaining capital funds should be allocated to regions in proportion to their weighted populations.

The formula approach to resource allocation -- criticisms and implementation

In this section we will provide a short survey of the criticisms that have been levelled against the reports on resource allocation and then consider the implementation of the proposals contained in the RAWP, SHARE, SCRAW and PARR reports. Most of the critical literature is aimed at RAWP, the first report to appear. Whilst it is clear that the authors of SHARE, SCRAW and PARR benefited from the debate that followed the publication of the RAWP report, some of the points raised are still relevant to all the reports.

Criticism

(*1*) *The exclusion of Family Practitioner Services* One defect of the allocation formulae is the exclusion of the primary care, Family Practitioner Services (FPS). This is because of the independent contractor status of the physicians and other professionals in this sector. Whilst the RAWP report recognises the seriousness of this omission and recommends research into the interaction of this sector with the rest of the NHS, SHARE and PARR take the view that the level of provision of these services is determined by demand and so full funding is appropriate. However, the spatial distribution of general practitioners is very unequal[8] and therefore the logic of the formula allocation approach would favour the inclusion of the primary care sector. Moreover, there exists a clear incentive at present, for the hospital services to shift costs onto the FPS where cash limits do not apply.

The exclusion of the primary care services may lead to an inequitable distribution of and an inefficient use of resources but the nature of the contract between the NHS and FPS professionals may make it difficult to include this sector in the resource allocation formula. (All FPS professionals have independent contractor status with the NHS, i.e. they are self-employed and not employees of the NHS.)

(2) *The use of SMRs as morbidity indicators* The main technical criticisms of the RAWP formula related to the use of SMRs and the calculation of cross-boundary flows. One objection to the use of SMRs that is relevant to all the reports is that SMRs are inappropriate as indicators of morbidity.[9] However, this argument is only supported by the low correlation between SMRs and other suggested indicators of morbidity, such as GP consultation rates and self--reported sickness from the General Household Survey. No attempt has been made to show that these alternatives are more suitable indicators of relative need, particularly with respect to non-psychiatric in-patient services, the largest part of the allocation to be affected by the use of SMRs. A more valid criticism, made by Barr and Logan, relates to the assumption of a linear relationship between SMRs and relative need. As the true relationship has not yet been established, it is difficult to see any alternative to this simple assumption.

The use of condition specific SMRs below regional level has been criticised.[10] The RAWP report recognised that fluctuations might occur because of the small numbers involved at sub-regional level and suggested that a ten-year data base would eliminate this problem. However, a twenty-year simulation exercise carried out by Geary failed to 'predict' the true value of the SMR. These data are clearly suspect at this level and this supports the decision of SHARE, SCRAW, and PARR to use only overall SMRs.

(3) *The problem of cross-boundary flows* The handling of cross-boundary flows is another area which is open to criticism. The RAWP method, in particular, has been criticised as it relies on converting net flows into population equivalents by reference to the national admission rate.[11] The accredited population will be over-estimated if the local admission rate is higher and vice versa. This is particularly serious if, as seems likely, well endowed regions are net importers and have high admission rates. A second criticism arises from the use of national average specialty costs by RAWP and SCRAW and hospital group average costs by SHARE and PARR. Buxton and Klein have argued that more complex, and therefore more costly, cases will cross boundaries,[12] and this seems to be confirmed by a study at St Mary's Hospital, Paddington.[13] This problem is solved for some regional specialties by separate allocations made in the SHARE, SCRAW and PARR reports and by the separate cost of cross-boundary flows introduced in the 1980/81 RAWP allocations, following the recommendations of the Advisory Group on Resource Allocation (AGRA).[14]

The long-term aim of RAWP is to eliminate the majority of cross-boundary flows between regions, as these are mainly caused by a lack of facilities. At this level, any distortions created by the formula will diminish. However, in Scotland, Wales and Northern Ireland and within the English regions substantial flows will remain and an exact financial compensation would require costly cross-accounting to be carried out. In purely economic terms, an incentive for low-cost areas and low-cost hospitals to import cases, which they treat more efficiently, benefits the NHS although it will have adverse effects on the geographic distribution of resources. Dudley and Klein have suggested that increased patient mobility should be considered as a method of achieving equal access to services regardless of their geographic location, i.e. perhaps Regions and Districts should 'buy in' services from neighbouring areas with excess capacity rather than have their own services in all treatment areas.[15]

(4) *London and 'centres of excellence'* A substantial part of the RAWP literature has been aimed at a defence of the high allocations made in the past to the London Areas.[16] It is argued that an allowance should be made for the non-teaching costs of teaching hospitals because of the need to maintain the national and international 'centres of excellence' in London, and also that higher regional labour costs should be taken into account. In order to maintain staff levels, the Thames areas pay higher than average wage rates by making appointments at higher grades on the salary scale. The first problem does not affect SHARE, SCRAW and PARR, as these reports recommend that non-teaching costs should be allowed for, but the problem of grade drift is likely to be relevant in parts of Scotland, Wales and Northern Ireland. A 'market forces' weighting has been devised by the AGRA[17] and was implemented in the 1980/81 RAWP allocations but the 'centres of excellence' problem has not yet been resolved and could be complicated by the ambiguity of the term.

(5) *The use of historic (past) expenditure patterns* Another criticism is the use of historic expenditure patterns in weighting the service areas.[18] The change in emphasis away from acute hospital services in England has been laid out in the Department of Health and Social Security Priorities document[19] and a similar change in priorities may take place in Scotland, Wales and Northern Ireland. The substitution of the Priorities weightings into the RAWP formula made only marginal changes in the allocations,[20] but the use of historic weightings will tend to work against attempts to try and change established patterns of care.

(6) *Capital allocations* Finally, there are the problems associated with the allocation of capital resources. The value of the NHS stock of capital and equipment is unknown and current accounting practices ignore both depreciation and interest payments. This latter factor means that capital is 'free' to users: it involves no opportunity costs.

The impact of the capital allocation proposed by RAWP has been less immediate than the revenue proposals, with only a small part of the total budget being devoted to redistribution. Most of the available capital is allocated according to the weighted populations, so the criticisms of the RAWP revenue formula are equally relevant. Buxton and Klein[21] and Forbes[22] discuss the specific problems associated with the RAWP capital valuation, such as the failure to take account of mislocated or inappropriate capital stocks and the level of aggregation used. Forbes has also presented a method, similar to RAWP, for the redistribution of Scotland's capital resources.[23] It is clear that in order to achieve an equitable distribution of health resources in Scotland, Wales and Northern Ireland, capital allocation cannot be ignored. However, because of their relative sizes, the RAWP proposals for sub-regional allocation may be more relevant to Scotland, Wales and Northern Ireland. In order for sufficient capital to be available for major schemes, the RAWP report proposed that the historic capital stock deficit should only be used to determine priorities for capital. If this approach were to be adopted in Scotland, Wales and Northern Ireland further consideration would have to be given to the extent to which cross-boundary flows were to be eliminated. The criteria used to allocate capital in all parts of the NHS is unsatisfactory and has not been helped greatly by RAWP and the other formulae. Rational allocation can only be achieved if competing authorities have to bid for resources (like in a market) and pay the costs associated with the use of such resources (i.e. they meet depreciation and interest charges).

Implementation

(*1*) *RAWP* The RAWP allocation formula was the first to be introduced, with the RHA allocations for 1976/77 based on the interim report and those from 1977/78 onwards based on the final report. The implementation of RAWP is based on incremental growth rates, determined by each region's distance above or below its target allocation. These target allocations have been subject to change because of modifications to the RAWP formula, changes in the data base and population changes. Table 6.1 compares the situation of the regions in 1977/78 and 1981/82. All the regions have moved closer to their target positions, although Oxford has gone from an above target allocation to a below target allocation. This is because of the upward movement in Oxford's target share, mainly because of increases in the region's population.

The effect of RAWP on capital allocation is examined in Table 6.2. The first two columns show the capital stock deficit or surplus and the

Table 6.1 The effects of RAWP on revenue allocations (England)

	1977/78			*1981/82*		
Regional Health Authority	*Percentage share in main revenue allocation (excluding SHIFT)*	*Target share percentage*	*Distance from target percentage of actual allocation*	*Percentage share in main revenue allocation (excluding SIFT)*	*Target share percentage*	*Distance from target as percentage of actual allocation*
Trent	8.38	9.23	−10.14	8.64	9.22	−6.71
North Western	8.71	9.66	−10.91	9.06	9.62	−6.14
East Anglia	3.58	3.77	−5.31	3.67	3.88	−5.56
Northern	6.38	7.02	−10.03	6.60	6.94	−5.21
Wessex	5.18	5.51	−6.37	5.25	5.50	−4.78
South Western	6.36	6.68	−5.03	6.44	6.75	−4.74
West Midlands	10.06	10.68	−6.16	10.30	10.70	−3.89
Yorkshire	7.33	7.65	−4.37	7.41	7.68	−3.71
Oxford	4.27	3.98	+ 6.79	4.21	4.26	−1.18
Mersey	5.51	5.72	−3.81	5.48	5.50	−0.30
SW Thames	7.19	6.75	+6.12	6.97	6.57	+ 5.67
NE Thames	9.46	8.17	+ 13.64	9.06	8.26	+8.85
SE Thames	9.03	7.91	+ 12.40	8.65	7.89	+8.87
NW Thames	8.55	7.27	+ 14.97	8.25	7.23	+12.33

Sources: Department of Health and Social Security figures: RCPIC 22 February 1977 and circular RRA 16/2 26 February 1981.

Table 6.2 The effects of RAWP on capital allocations (England)

Regional Health Authority	*Deficit (–) or surplus (+) in capital stock, per head of population (March 1977 capital stock)* (1)	*Weighted population share for capital allocations 1976/77* (1)	*Percentage share in capital allocations* 1977/78 (2)	1981/82 (3)
North Western	–16.54	9.49	8.58	12.59
Wessex	–11.42	5.78	7.33	7.02
Trent	–7.72	9.58	15.37	9.74
West Midlands	–6.75	10.75	6.67	9.72
Yorkshire	–5.72	7.82	7.14	8.27
Northern	–4.13	6.83	7.06	7.27
South Western	–1.16	6.64	5.55	6.33
SE Thames	+0.84	7.96	4.66	6.20
East Anglia	+5.74	3.79	5.20	5.20
SW Thames	+8.27	6.40	6.83	5.38
Oxford	+11.24	4.42	5.78	4.13
NE Thames	+13.54	7.84	5.82	7.21
NW Thames	+16.28	7.14	5.08	5.53
Mersey	+17.53	5.54	8.93	5.42

Sources: (1) Department of Health and Social Security, *Sharing Resources for Health in England*, report of the Resource Allocation Working Party, London: HMSO, 1976.
(2) *British Medical Journal* vol. i, 1977, p. 780.
(3) Department of Health and Social Security, personal communication.

weighted population shares, as calculated in the RAWP report.[24] These two factors should determine the capital allocation. However, the 1977/78 allocations were dominated by commitments that had already been made. Although the population figures will have been revised slightly, the 1981/82 allocations show that with the exception of West Midlands and East Anglia, Regional Authorities with a capital stock deficit received higher allocations than their weighted population would indicate and regions with a surplus received lower allocations. Some progress is being made in reducing capital stock deficits, but the pace of change will be determined by several factors, most importantly by the level of resources available.

(2) *SHARE* The SHARE formula has been used as the basis for revenue allocations since 1978/79. The redistribution is being achieved very gradually with the 1978/79 allocations being designed to achieve one-tenth of the total redistribution, i.e. it is aimed at reaching equality in ten years, subject to the proviso that no allocation is reduced in real terms.[25] Also, a system of banking and borrowing has been introduced: allocated money that the Health Boards are unable to spend is being used to smooth over difficulties for other Boards. Compensating variations will be made in the future.[26]

Table 6.3 compares the position of the Health Boards in 1977/78, before SHARE was implemented, with the position in 1981/82. The range of the divergence from targets has been reduced and some of the Boards are nearer to their target positions. The movement of some Boards away from their target allocations is attributable to the revision of targets rather than to any failure to increase or reduce the allocations, as appropriate. The interpretation of these changes is further complicated by the application of cash limits, whereby overspending in any year is deducted from the following year's allocation and 1% of any underspending is carried forward.

(3) *SCRAW* The method of applying the SCRAW formula to the revenue allocations is different from RAWP and SHARE. The relative positions of the health authorities are only used as guidelines for the allocation of those growth funds set aside for equalisation. Total available growth funds are determined centrally and allocated between revenue consequences of capital schemes (RCCS), various non-capital developments and equalisation. Table 6.4 shows the results of the SCRAW formula allocations for 1976/77 and 1980/81, which were used as the basis for growth fund allocations in 1977/78 and 1981/82. In both of these cases, and in each of the intervening years, the Steering Committee has recommended that available equalisation funds should be

Table 6.3 The effects of the SHARE allocations (Scotland)

Health Board	*1977/78* Percentage share of revenue allocation (1)	Target share (percentage) (2)	Distance from target as a percentage of actual allocation	*1981/82* Percentage share of revenue allocation (1)	Target share (percentage) (1)	Distance from target as a percentage of actual allocation
Ayrshire and Arran	4.32	5.81	– 34.49	4.70	5.75	– 22.34
Islands	0.92	1.15	– 25.00	1.06	1.24	– 16.98
Borders	1.40	1.41	– 0.71	1.42	1.62	– 14.08
Fife	4.55	4.74	– 4.18	4.67	5.15	– 10.28
Forth Valley	4.54	4.75	– 4.63	4.64	4.92	– 6.03
Grampian	8.63	8.76	– 1.51	8.72	9.12	– 4.59
Lanarkshire	7.90	7.96	– 0.76	8.06	8.41	– 4.34
Dumfries and Galloway	2.50	2.66	– 6.40	2.57	2.64	– 2.72
Argyll and Clyde	7.12	7.29	– 2.39	7.31	7.43	– 1.64
Highland	3.73	3.65	+ 2.14	3.75	3.73	+ 0.53
Lothian	16.50	15.90	+ 3.64	16.16	15.48	+ 4.21
Greater Glasgow	27.59	27.14	+ 1.63	27.06	25.46	+ 5.91
Tayside	10.32	8.78	+ 14.92	9.88	9.05	+ 8.40

Sources: (1) Scottish Office, Finance Division, personal communications
(2) Scottish Home and Health Department *Annual Report*, Cmnd 7237, Edinburgh: HMSO, 1977.

Table 6.4 Application of the SCRAW revenue formula (Wales)

	1976/77			1980/81		
	Percentage share of basic revenue allocation[a]	*Target share (percentage)*	*Distance from target as a percentage of basic allocation*[a]	*Percentage share of basic revenue allocation*[a]	*Target share (percentage)*	*Distance from target as a percentage of basic allocation*[a]
Dyfed	10.77	11.73	– 8.91	10.71	11.75	– 9.71
West Glamorgan	13.09	15.06	– 15.05	13.62	14.59	– 7.12
Mid Glamorgan	17.90	18.07	– 0.95	17.62	18.12	– 2.84
Gwynedd	8.12	8.15	– 0.37	7.84	7.91	– 0.89
Clwyd	13.37	12.81	+ 4.19	13.12	12.98	+ 1.07
Powys	2.85	2.36	+ 17.19	2.80	2.76	+ 1.43
Gwent	15.31	15.73	– 2.74	15.95	15.14	+ 5.08
South Glamorgan	18.59	16.09	+ 13.45	18.33	16.75	+ 8.62

Note: [a]Hospital and community services revenue less earmarked sums for psychiatric hospitals, regional and sub-regional specialities and teaching allowance.

Sources: Welsh Office, *Report of the Steering Committee on Resource Allocation in Wales*, Cardiff, HMSO, 1977;
Welsh Office, *The Distribution of Resources to Health Authorities in Wales, Fifth Report of the Steering Committee* Cardiff: HMSO, 1981.

allocated to Dyfed and West Glamorgan. Changes in the positions of the other health authorities are the result of other growth fund allocations.

(4) *PARR* The PARR report was published at the end of 1978 and will be implemented in 1982/83. As Table 6.5 shows, the adjustments to allocations resulting from applying the formula are very minor. In view of the uncertainty about the accuracy and stability of the resource allocation procedure, the report recommends a cautious approach. The allocations to the Health Boards are to be determined by four factors: (i) the amount required to maintain present services updated for pay and price increases; (ii) RCCS; (iii) other earmarked allocations; and (iv) a minimum growth allocation to meet the requirements of a changing population. Any additional funds available would then be used for equalisation.

Table 6.5 Revenue allocations in Ulster

Health and Social Services Board	*Adjusted notional share* (%)	*Present allocation* (%)	*Adjustment required* (%)	*Adjustment as a percentage of present allocation*
Eastern	54.4	54.5	−0.1	−0.2
Northern	16.6	15.9	+ 0.7	+ 4.3
Southern	14.4	14.9	−0.5	−3.0
Western	14.6	14.7	−0.1	−0.7

Source: Department of Health and Social Services, *Proposals for the Allocation of Revenue Resources for Health and Personal Social Services*, Report of the Working Group on Revenue Resource Allocations to Health and Social Services Boards in Northern Ireland, 1978, Table 9B.

Inequality in the distribution of health care resources

In the preceding sections, the resource allocation procedures of the NHS have been analysed. The *ad hoc* (last year's budget plus *x*% for inflation, *y*% for growth, and *z*% to mitigate any scandals of a politically sensitive nature) budget allocation procedures which characterised the first twenty years of the NHS have been largely replaced by explicit allocation formulae whose characteristics differ in one part of the United Kingdom as from another. This section examines some remaining problems and policy issues.

The objective of these allocation formulae is to equalise the allocation of financial resources between regions. The allocations are weighted by 'need', which is proxied by standardised mortality data as a measure of morbidity (because no adequate direct measures of morbidity exist). As was pointed out earlier, SMRs may not be correlated with morbidity rates and, even if they are, there is no reason to suppose that this correlation is linear. These problems indicate the magnitude of ignorance about the prevalence and incidence of disease in the United Kingdom. The epidemiological base for planning and policy analysis is poor at present. A great deal of basic epidemiological research is required before the logic of the planning targets articulated in RAWP, SHARE, SCRAW and PARR can be analysed thoroughly. Until this research is completed, the appropriateness of using SMRs will be unknown.

Even if mortality data are good proxies for morbidity, increased financial allocations to deprived regions may not reduce mortality differences between the regions. The first problem is that while the area health authorities in England, and their counterparts elsewhere, are directed to apply RAWP criteria at the local level, they may do so in an imperfect manner. Forsyth and Varley have shown that allocations at the local level have been defective when viewed from the RAWP perspective and thus, despite the flow of increased resources to the North-West of England, services on the ground have not improved in some areas.[27] Whilst the process of reallocation from the centre to the regions has been able to withstand opposition from losing regions, various institutional forces may make implementation more difficult at the local level. All these forces, be they doctors, nurses, ancillary workers, local populations, politicians or bureaucrats, are self-interested and will work to maintain their allocations when faced by deprivation. Further, the reorganisation of the NHS in 1982, with the creation of nearly 200 districts and the advocacy of decentralisation, may bring with it less central willingness and ability to redistribute.

Secondly, even if the RAWP-type allocations are applied at subregional levels, there is no guarantee that resources will be allocated to the 'neediest' members of the community. This aspect of the RAWP process is particularly important in the context of social class inequalities in health. The problem was recognised by the members of the first SCRAW:

> The attention of the Steering Committee has also been drawn to evidence that the use made of different parts of the health service varies with social class, generally in the direction of less use being made by people at the lower end of the social scale. The argument presented suggests that it is not enough to assume that services will necessarily be used by those who most require them; authorities should aim to ensure that services are appropriately deployed and are really used by those in greatest need.[28]

In general, there has been no monitoring of the effects of resource reallocation on the services received by communities at the local level. However, more attention may be focused on this issue following the publication of the Black Report on inequalities in health.[29] Amongst other recommendations, the authors suggested that a special health and social development programme should be experimented with in the ten areas of England with the highest SMRs. The Secretary of State for Health and Social Services rejected these recommendations and pointed out that the areas of greatest need identified by the Black Report are receiving areas under the RAWP formula.[30]

Given the lack of information that exists both about the application of RAWP criteria at local levels and about the deployment of additional resources, this response is unlikely to remedy such inequalities. Now that the RAWP process has been established, it is time to evaluate its effect at local levels, to examine whether more sensitive indicators, such as social class or income, could be used at sub-regional levels and to consider whether less discretion should be given to regions in determining local allocations.

The final reason why new financial allocations may not reduce regional disparities in health status is because increased finance, even if spent on improved health care, may not always improve health status. Even the Royal Commission on the NHS seems to have got the message that increased inputs (of finance, manpower or other resources) do not always and everywhere lead to increased outputs of 'good health'.[31] Perhaps the most important strands of this debate are the arguments of Cochrane, that most therapies have not been scientifically evaluated,[32] and McKeown, that the main cause of the decline in mortality during the 1838–1938 period and beyond was improvements in nutrition and not advances in medicine.[33]

The implication of this line of argument is that it may be pointless to equalise resources between regions if those regions spend their health resources in an inefficient manner. The increased availability of resources in the Trent and Northern regions of England may not lead to improved health status there. Similarly relatively less resources in the Thames regions may not reduce the health status of their populations. The links, if any, between inputs and outputs in health care are poorly understood and require careful evaluation and monitoring. The effects of RAWP and the other formulae on the efficiency with which scarce resources are used is not clear and requires careful monitoring.

Conclusion

The allocation formulae devised to redistribute health care resources in England, Scotland, Wales and Northern Ireland were described in the first section of this chapter. Some criticisms of the various elements of the formulae were presented in the first part of the second section, followed by an examination of the effects of implementing these formulae. The concentration of criticism on particular details of the allocation formulae has tended to deflect attention from other issues, such as the kind of equality that the RAWP process is attempting to achieve, which are potentially more important. The terms of reference of the RAWP were to devise a method of resource allocation that would achieve 'a pattern of distribution responsive objectively, equitably and efficiently to relative need.'[34]

The working Party chose to interpret this as equal financial allocations for populations at equal risk, and the authors of the subsequent reports have followed this lead. This begs the question of whether equal financial allocations lead to an equal supply of health services and whether equal health care services lead to equal health status, either of which could be taken as alternative objectives for redistribution. The result is that several policy issues concerning equal access to health care remain untouched and these were reviewed in the third section. The setting of precise objectives and the monitoring of outcomes have been, and continue to be, weaknesses in the policy-making process. In terms of their effect on the unequal distribution of financial allocations, the resource allocation formulae have been successful. Their effects on the allocation of real resources and on differences in health status remain unexplored. RAWP and the associated formulae are policy innovations which, like so many health care policies in the UK and elsewhere, require evaluation but have been deprived of this necessary requisite of efficient resource allocation.

Notes

1. Ministry of Health, *A Hospital Plan for England and Wales*, Cmnd 1604, London: HMSO, 1962.
2. Department of Health and Social Security, *Regional Resource Allocation Formula*, First interim report of the Resource Allocation Working Party, London: HMSO, 1975.
3. Department of Health and Social Security, *Sharing Resources for Health in England*, report of the Resource Allocation Working Party, London: HMSO, 1976.
4. Scottish Home and Health Department, *Scottish Health Authorities Revenue Equalisation*, report of the Working Party on Revenue Resource Allocation, Edinburgh: HMSO, 1977.
5. Welsh Office, *Report of the Steering Committee on Resource Allocation in Wales*, Cardiff: HMSO, 1977.
6. Department of Health and Social Services, *Proposals for the Allocation of Revenue Resources for Health and Personal Social Services*, report of the Working Group on Revenue Resource Allocations to Health and Social Services Boards in Northern Ireland, 1978.
7. This is based on a study of teaching hospitals summarised in A. J. Culyer, J. Wiseman, M. F. Drummond and P. A. West, 'What Accounts for the Higher Costs of Teaching Hospitals?', *Social and Economic Administration*, Vol. 12, no. 1, 1978, pp. 20–30.

8. M. H. Cooper and A. J. Culyer, 'An Economic Survey of the Nature and Intent of the British National Health Service', *Social Science and Medicine*, Vol. 5, 1971, pp. 1–13, and J. T. Hart, 'The inverse care law', *Lancet*, Vol. i, 1971, pp. 405–12.
9. A. Barr and R. F. L. Logan, 'Policy alternatives for resource allocation', *Lancet*, Vol. i, 1977, pp. 994–7, and D. P. Forster, 'Mortality, Morbidity and Resource Allocation', *Lancet*, Vol. i, 1977, pp. 997–8.
10. K. Geary, 'Technical deficiencies in RAWP', *British Medical Journal*, Vol. i, 1977, p. 1367, and S. R. Palmer, P. A. West and P. Dodd, 'Randomness in the RAWP formula: the reliability of mortality data in the allocation of National Health Service revenue', *Journal of Epidemiology and Community Health*, Vol. 34, no. 3, pp. 212–16.
11. S. J. Senn and H. Shaw, 'Resource allocation. Some problems in applying the national formula to area and district revenue allocations', *Journal of Epidemiology and Community Health*, Vol. 32, 1978, pp. 22–7.
12. M. J. Buxton and R. E. Klein, 'Allocating health resources. A commentary on the report of the RAWP', *Royal Commission on the National Health Services*, Research Paper No. 3, London: HMSO, 1978.
13. H. Lyons, 'Unless the sums are right the answers will be wrong', *Pulse*, 27 January 1979.
14. Department of Health and Social Security, *Report of the Advisory Group on Resource Allocation*, 1980.
15. H. A. F. Dudley, 'Loosening patient immobility', *Lancet*, Vol. i, 1977, pp. 1251–3, and R. E. Klein, 'Resource allocation', *Hospital and Health Services Review*, August 1977, pp. 280–4.
16. Sir F. A. Jones, 'The London hospitals scene', *British Medical Journal*, Vol. ii, 1976, pp. 1046–9, and W. F. Whimster, 'Personal View', *British Medical Journal*, Vol. ii, 1976, p. 1318.
17. DHSS, *Report of the Advisory Group on Resource Allocation.*
18. A. L. Creese, S. C. Darby, S. R. Palmer and D. L. Patrick, 'NHS priorities and RAWP', *British Medical Journal*, Vol. ii, 1978, pp. 1446–7.
19. Department of Health and Social Security, *Priorities for Health and Personal Social Services in England*, London: HMSO, 1976.
20. Creese *et al.*, 'NHS priorities and RAWP'.
21. 'Allocating health resources'.
22. J. F. Forbes, *Capital Valuation and the Health Services: A Review of Theory and Practice*, University of Aberdeen Health Economics Research Unit, Discussion paper no. 01/79, 1979.
23. J. F. Forbes, *Sharing Health Service Capital Resources in Scotland*, University of Aberdeen Health Economics Research Unit, Discussion Paper no. 02/79, 1979.
24. DHSS, *Sharing Resources for Health in England.*
25. Scottish Home and Health Department, *Health Services in Scotland Report for 1978*, Cmnd 7607, Edinburgh: HMSO, 1979.
26. House of Commons Hansard, 18 January 1878, 250/1.
27. G. Forsyth and R. Varley, Resource Allocation Subregionally: the Impact in the North-West RHA, mimeo, 1978.
28. Welsh Office, *Report of the Steering Committee on Resource Allocation in Wales*, p. 63.
29. Department of Health and Social Security, *Inequalities in Health. Report of a research working group* (The Black Report), 1980.
30. 'Commentary from Westminster: Mr Jenkin on the Black Report', *Lancet*, Vol. i, 1981, pp. 735–6.
31. Royal Commission on the National Health Service (Chairman Sir Alec Merrison), *Report*, Cmnd 7616, London: HMSO, 1979.
32. A. L. Cochrane, *Effectiveness and Efficiency: random reflections on Health Services*, London: Nuffield Provincial Hospital Trust, 1972.
33. T. McKeown, *The Modern Rise of Population*, London: Edward Arnold, 1976.
34. DHSS, *Sharing Resources for Health in England*, p. 5.

7 The 'Auld Enemy': comparing different systems for delivering the personal social services and juvenile Justice in Great Britain

Gilbert Smith[1]

Introduction

The term 'comparative social administration' is most often taken to refer to the study of the major services of the welfare state in Britain, in relation to those services which fulfil approximately equivalent functions within other countries. Frequent comparitors are the USA and countries of Western Europe although these are by no means the only examples. There also exist, however, *within* Britain, differences which may repay comparative examination. Although these differences are sometimes glossed over, especially in textbooks, they in fact offer policy research a significant advantage, for one of the major problems of comparative research across nations is that there are so many cultural, financial, linguistic, political and other differences that it is extremely difficult to isolate those variables that are of policy significance. Within Britain the task of using a comparative exercise to identify differences in the causes and consequences of various policies and administrative arrangements may be a little easier because, for example, there is a common constitution, for the most part a common language, and so on. This paper is especially about policy related research into the structure and functioning of the personal social services and the organisation of juvenile justice.[2] In particular it deals with the question of how those differences in service provision which exist as between Scotland, on the one hand, and England and Wales on the other, may be turned to advantage in the design of comparative research.[3]

In outline, the paper will run along the following path. Frequently the differences which are to be found in legislation, the administrative framework, personnel, categories and styles of service, and in other matters, are regarded by research workers as insignificant, inconvenient or methodologically embarrassing. By reviewing briefly some of the major parallels and divergencies in social work and related services between north and south Britain it is possible to suggest research which may be conducted to capitalise upon this variation.[4] In general terms that is really not so very difficult. Indeed it is rather obvious that comparative social work research within Britain is potentially very fruitful. The puzzling question is not so much what research could be done as why there is currently such a paucity of research of this kind, why its merits have not been taken more seriously, and why it is therefore now necessary to champion its attractions. The point is that little purpose is to be served by suggesting comparisons between social work and social services departments, between juvenile courts and children's panels or whatever, unless we have some grasp of why these topics have remained neglected to date.

It will be an argument of the final part of the paper that although there are undoubtedly conceptual and methodological complications in designing research which spans the Tweed, the major barriers are nevertheless institutional rather than intellectual. It follows that the effort of initiating comparative research in the personal social services lies as much in the realm of funding, staffing, organising, publishing, disseminating and implementing research, and in its highly political connotations, as it does in *a priori* conceptual analysis. This is not to dispute the importance of formulating sound questions for much research founders because the central issues have been inadequately construed. This paper will consider briefly some issues of research design and problem formulation but will also review some of the factors that seem to have inhibited research, whatever its specific focus, that compares the different systems of social work and juvenile justice within Britain.

Before embarking on that task, however, there are at least two pitfalls to be avoided, and it is wise to mention these dangers at an early stage. The first point is that prospects for research in this field are not bright if the case for comparative studies is seen as an instance of special pleading from the Celtic fringe, or a symptom of the general Scottish feeling that the English do not take them seriously. Both Scottish politicians and civil servants in the Scottish Office will know that this feeling is by no means confined to the terraces of Hampden Park. The insensitivity of DHSS and Home Office opposite numbers on aspects of Scottish legislation and administration is a frequent source of irritation and although this subject is often talked about in a jocular fashion it is not unreasonable to conclude that there is here an important factor cementing departmental boundaries and perpetuating the compartmentalised thinking which tends to pervade the machinery of policy-making in government. It is also true that students of social work and juvenile justice in Scotland are on occasions disappointed at the apparent lack of interest in their research. They complain too, perhaps legitimately, that academics south of the border are less well informed about Scottish legislation than is the reverse.[5] But the case for comparative research must rest not upon the importance of distinctly Scottish policy questions nor upon the merits of studying social work as opposed to social services departments, or the panel system as opposed to the juvenile court, nor upon the alleged neglect of data collected north of the border. The case must be that by studying both social work and social services departments, and both panels and juvenile courts, then it becomes possible to solve problems which it would otherwise be more difficult to solve. In the past, teams located neither north nor south of the border have not been very successful in either identifying or solving problems of that kind. In consequence, solutions that might have been revealed have remained clouded from view.

The second pitfall to be avoided is that of regarding the fundamental design problems of comparative research within Britain as unique. It is a presumption of this paper that the case for comparative research within Britain needs to be argued, but there is, of course, a sense in which all research is comparative. Although relatively little policy research follows a rigorous experimental approach the basic, if implicit, logic is invariably that of holding some factors constant, or otherwise controlling them, and allowing other factors to vary. The causes, consequences and desirability of the variations are then explored. The fundamental limitation of the case study, whatever the unit of the case, is that although it may be suggestive, the implications are limited because of the absence of comparison.

The significance of this rather general point for the present paper is that in consequence we are bound to be precise about exactly which aspects of juvenile justice or social work we are seeking to compare. There are, after all, major differences within both north and south Britain which allow many questions to be studied. In social work in Scotland for instance there are significant differences in the budget of departments (as between Strathclyde and the Western Isles), in their geographical size (as between Glasgow and Orkney), in economic prosperity and decline (as between Aberdeen and Dumfries), in the proportions of trained workers, in the official recorded incidence of a range of primary problems, in the internal structure of departments, in religious and cultural attitudes to welfare, as between Highland and Lowland Scotland, east and west coast, Gaelic and English speaking, and so on. It is important in stressing the utility of comparisons between north and south Britain that we should not presume the homogeneous nature of the personal social services within each area. Thus we encounter at a very early stage that problem which bedevils so much research in social work at the present time: the difficulty of knowing empirically what *are* the constituent practices of social work, although, as I have argued, it does seem that this difficulty is more manageable *within* the British context than when making broader international comparisons.

Comparative differences

Our starting point must be the existing important legal and administrative differences between the organisations of social work and juvenile justice, north and south of the border. Himsworth has provided material which is most helpful in grasping the statutory position (see Chapter 4 of this volume), but it may be useful to highlight one or two features of the legislation particularly relevant to social work and juvenile justice and present a summary statement of the main comparative differences. It will simplify this section of the paper if I make a few points in synoptic form.[6]

1. Social work in Britain in its present style is very much a product of the legal changes and administrative reorganisation which took place in the late 1960s and early 1970s.
2. These changes were accompanied by an expansion of social work both numerically, institutionally and, equally important, conceptually. That is, areas of provision within the welfare state and criminal justice system that had previously not necessarily been regarded as aspects of the personal social services were redefined as 'social work'.
3. This process in turn was accompanied by an ongoing debate about the nature of delinquency which led to important changes in the organisation of juvenile justice.
4. The outcomes of these changes were somewhat different in Scotland, from England and Wales.

The legislative basis for the English and Welsh social services departments is the 1970 Local Authority Social Services Act.[7] This brought together the previously separate Children's and Welfare departments in each local authority and established a single agency to provide, within each area, the vast majority of the personal social services including child care and guidance, some aspects of mental health, welfare of the elderly, the substantial home help service, and welfare services previously provided by some health and housing departments. Developments heralding this act can be traced to 1956 when the Ingleby Committee was appointed with terms of reference covering juvenile courts and preventive work with children[8] leading to an expanded role for the child care service in the 1963 Children and Young Person Act. Shortly afterwards, in 1965, the white paper *The Child, the Family, and the Young Offender* was published. Although its proposal for 'family courts' fell when the paper was withdrawn, to be replaced in 1968 by *Children in Trouble* which gained legislative form as the Children and Young Persons Act, 1969, the paper was particularly important in questioning the boundaries between social welfare, and juvenile justice as a primarily legal matter. The possibility of what in scientific research might be called a 'paradigm shift' in social work was also apparent in this report in the announcement of the government's intention to set up a committee to examine the structuring of the whole range of personal social services at the local authority level. This committee was to produce the *Report of the Committee on Local Authority and Allied Personal Social Services* (The Seebohm report) in 1968 and during 1971 social services departments were established in the south. The probation service in England and Wales retains separate functions although much of the work of probation with juveniles has been reformulated and placed within the ambit of officers of the social services department. Probation officers are inclined not to describe themselves as social workers.

Hall has documented in some detail the political aspects of this reorganisation in southern social work.[9] But in spite of the fact that the recommendations of the Seebohm report and its implementation have been extensively debated in the professional literature, usually from the standpoint of some particular interest group, there remains, some ten years after the passing of major legislation, a serious dearth of empirical research material which might serve as the basis for evaluating, comparing or even describing the practical activities of this group of social work agencies.[10] The state of research in this field is particularly unhealthy when we recall the firm comments of the Seebohm report:

> The personal social services are large-scale experiments in ways of helping those in need. It is both wasteful and irresponsible to set experiments in motion and omit to record and analyse what happens. (para 455).
>
> The planning of the personal social services cannot be undertaken successfully without the research which identifies emerging trends, assesses long-term repercussions, and estimates the character and dimension of future needs. (para 457).
>
> We cannot emphasise too strongly the part which research must play in the creation and maintenance of an effective family service. (para 473).[11]

The legislative basis for the Scottish social work departments is the Social Work (Scotland) Act 1968.[12] Its provisions were foreshadowed by the McBoyle Committee report on the *Prevention of Neglect of Children* which recommended that the services of separate local authority departments should be coordinated within a single 'family welfare service'. But the Act derives primarily from the report of the Kilbrandon Committee *Children and Young Persons, Scotland.* This report began with the familiar problem of public concern at the rising level of officially recorded juvenile delinquency and much of its discussions concerned the reorganisation of the diverse forms of the Scottish juvenile court.[13] Sections of the report, however, also dealt with the concomitant reorganisation of social work which would be required to provide personal social services in support of the new organisation. This consideration took the form of recommending the establishment of social education departments which were to become the present social work departments in each local authority area. Thus the present form of administration in local authority social work grew out of a concern to strengthen the system of delinquency control although it may well be argued that in practice the pattern of influence has been just the reverse and social work has colonised juvenile justice. Certainly important features of both the children's panel system and the personal social services north of the border derive from the interaction of the two. While changes in the juvenile courts and the child care service were contemporaries in south Britain the organisational links in the process of change were much closer in the north.

In *Social Work and the Community* the government broadly accepted Kilbrandon's recommendations although, as I have mentioned, the 'education' department became a 'social work' department, and the white paper certainly does not convey the impression that the operation of the personal social services should be subservient to the requirements of juvenile justice. Within central government the Social Work Services Group was created within the Scottish Education Department to oversee the new legislation and its implementation. As in the South the act brought together the services of welfare and child care. (Medical social work was included at a later date.) But in Scotland the probation service, too, became a component of 'generic' social work. Section 12 of the act also has no direct southern counterpart. This section lays upon every local authority the duty 'to promote social welfare by making available advice, guidance and assistance on such a scale as may be appropriate for their area', and allows that, 'Assistance given in kind or in cash to, or in respect of, persons under this section may be given unconditionally. . . .' The new directors of social work assumed their powers in Autumn 1969 and the children's hearings became operative in spring 1971.

There exists no published study on the politics of the creation of juvenile justice and the organisation of social work in Scotland to compare with Hall.[15] Such a study would explain how social work successfully retained conceptual and administrative independence from the control of education and the health service. It would explain why some sections of the probation service were unsuccessful in defending their separate service and sections of the judiciary could not prevent the advent of the children's panels. It would also detail the origins of section 12. Data on the functioning of social work departments are likewise sparse. Rees studied clients from two agencies in Scotland one of which was a local authority department, but the main interest of this research is in professional–client interaction rather than in specifically policy questions,[16] as is also the case in Voysey which touches on Scottish social work.[17] This comment is not, of course, a criticism and the approaches are not separate but, as I shall go on to suggest, research workers with Scottish material may be discouraged from presenting their data within the framework of comparative policy debate. Blaxter's study of the network of agencies concerned with disability contains data on the relationships between social work departments and related services.[18] Stevenson reports a study conducted jointly by a Scottish and English based team of research workers.[19] Jackson and Valencia draw upon their experience of research on the use of section 12 of the Scottish legislation to provide financial aid through social work.[20]

The literature on northern juvenile justice is somewhat richer. Curran reviews this literature.[21] He combines material from several studies and reanalyses secondary data, but he is inclined to over-emphasise the significance of some of the smaller studies. There are several thoughtful reviews of the system some of which draw upon empirical research.[22] Bruce and Spencer's book arose out of a research project although little of the empirical material is available.[23] The discussion in Morris and McIsacc goes considerably beyond their data.[24] Martin, Fox and Murray is the most recent substantial research report.[25] Martin and Murray[26] and Brown and Bloomfield[27] are contrasting collections of readings. The former contains papers written from the perspective of the various parties involved in the system, and the latter places what contributors see as the issues raised by the panel system within the context of broader social and legal debates. Parsloe offers an ambitious comparative survey of juvenile justice systems both within Britain and in America, but the book highlights the problems of attempting broad comparisons without data geared to a particular problem and a specific difference. The basis of claims that

> The children's hearing is governed by the concepts of a welfare approach. (p. 175).

or The aim [of hearings] is to have an informal friendly discussion and, with such aims, procedural rules are out of place. (p. 176).

or Panel members are not responsible for protecting the public. (p. 177).

are entirely problematic.[28] The difficulty here is that, as with so much of this literature,[29] in the absence of original empirical research, impressionistic material, personal bias and the statements of government reports, of one kind or another, tend to fill the gap. In consequence much discussion is either polemical, in the form of radical criticisms of the system or a complacent account reflecting the ideals of an 'official view', or else reflects individual interpretations of what the underlying principles of systems, which depart from the juvenile court, are supposed to be and mean.

To summarise, then, I have been seeking in this first part of the paper simply to identify major differences in social work and juvenile justice within Britain which might serve to focus comparative research. A first, if somewhat pessimistic, conclusion must be this. Since 1968 there has been published insufficient original empirical research to allow us to identify, independent of government sources,[30] actual concrete differences in the practical performance of the social work and juvenile justice systems in north and south Britain. That is not to say that there are no differences. But it is very difficult to be precise about what they are, and I have already concurred with the view that this kind of precision is a pre-requisite to comparative research. The second conclusion is that we are therefore limited in our starting points to legal and broad administrative variations, and differences within the policy debates upon which these legal and administrative structures are based.

I have pointed to some comparative differences of this type. Primarily these are:

1. The probation service. England and Wales retain a probation service distinct from that of the remainder of the personal social services and separate from local authority control. In Scotland probation became a local authority responsibility in 1971 and is administered as an integral part of social work departments. Professionals are trained as 'generic' workers without formal specialisation.[31]

2. The system of children's panels. England and Wales retain a juvenile court, albeit modified by the Children and Young Persons Act 1969. In Scotland the Sheriff court continues to play a part in juvenile justice but an essentially court based system has been replaced by the children hearings. Apart from the different relationship between welfare authorities and the judiciary, the system embodies selected lay volunteers and an official called the Reporter, in crucial decision-making roles. Neither panel members nor the Reporter have comparable counterparts in the South.

3. Financial aid and the promotion of welfare. Under section 12 of the Social Work (Scotland) Act 1968 Scottish local authorities possess powers and responsibilities that are distinct from those accruing to social services departments under the Local Authority Social Services Act 1970, although related powers in the South are retained under the Children and Young Persons Act 1963.

4. Central government administration. There are differences in the way in which responsibilities are assigned at central government level. In the south the personal social services fall to the Department of Health and Social Security, the Home Office and the Health and Social Work Department of the Welsh Office. In Scotland the Social Work Services Group

lies within the Scottish Education Department. DHSS social security functions extend to Scotland and adult criminal justice is the responsibility of the Home and Health Department within the Scottish Office.[32]

5. The history of legal and aministrative change. The history of the creation of social work and social services departments is different. It is not as straightforward as saying that Kilbradon was the equivalent of Seebohm in Scotland. Particularly important was the fact that in the North the debates about 'generic' social work, on the one hand, and about 'punishment', 'treatment' and 'justice' in relation to juvenile delinquency on the other, were linked more directly in legal and administrative terms. The current organisational differences represent different outcomes to major conceptual and policy debates, and political battles. It is also the case that the achievements of social work in ensuring that its aspirations to professional autonomy were matched by institutional autonomy, especially in remaining independence of health and education, are all the more significant in Scotland where many of the services prior to 1969 were in an elementary state in comparison to the south.

Comparative differences as a problem

Any attempt to describe or analyse the personal social services and juvenile justice in Britain should clearly take account of at least the more significant of these differences between North and South. Yet, apparently, social scientists find this to be a problem, and we encounter in the literature, typically, one of four reactions.

The first reaction to the problem is simply to *ignore* it. It is particularly frustrating for those teaching comparative social administration or teaching in Scotland that this is often the approach of standard texts.[33] Marshall for example makes no mention of Kilbrandon, children's panels or social work departments,[34] and the same is true of Brown in spite of the fact that the book is titled *Introduction to Social Administration in Britain.*[35] But researchers likewise tend to think of England (or Scotland) as the unit of analysis, whether or not this best serves the purposes of the investigation. Comparative differences are ignored as a resource.

The second reaction to the problem is to note, but *dismiss* it. Marsh's *Introducing Social Policy* contains a particularly blatant illustration of this approach when the author writes of

> . . . Britain (and that means basically England and Wales because Scotland differs in some respects in its methods of provision of some social services) . . .[36]

Directly relevant to the interests of this paper, Sainsbury's *The Personal*

Social Services is also a typical example of the way in which Scottish material is treated much more briefly as a kind of addendum, certainly giving the impression (perhaps unintended) that the differences are not really all that significant.[37]

A third reaction to the problem of the differences involves a seemingly quite deliberate attempt to *minimise* any impression of variation between north and south Britain. This reaction is particularly characteristic of the literature reporting research that was carried out in Scotland and is a stance which is apparently adopted (probably perfectly rationally) in anticipation of the criticism that the work is parochial and of limited significance. Jackson and Valencia is one example.[38] The authors have been involved in research concerning financial aid through social work for a number of years and collected their data in Scottish social work departments. Much of the book draws on material from many sources but the chapter on decision-making is based upon their own investigations. Nevertheless the introduction explains that 'Most of the discussion will be based on British material'.[39] Now I am not at all suggesting that the conclusions of this book are misleading or that the data are analysed in illigitimate ways. I am simply pointing to the fact that comparative differences in arrangements for financial aid in social work tend to be minimised rather than highlighted. It is worth quoting the objectives of the study in full:

> First, we shall examine the ways in which the financial aid responsibilities of social work departments overlap with similar responsibilities in other agencies. Second, we shall look at the way social workers make decisions on financial aid and at some of the factors that influence these decisions. Third, we shall speculate about the consequences of the decision made, for example, on the relationship of financial aid to the social work task.[40]

It would seem a positive advantage that there is variation between north and south Britain in factors associated with each of these issues. But that is not the approach.

Rees is another example.[41] I have mentioned that this study is based upon data about the interaction between clients and social workers located in two agencies in Scotland, one of them a local authority department. But the distinctive features of this context play no special part in the analysis or presentation of the material. The review of staff ideologies, for instance, does not place these ideas in the context of the particular policies that featured in the Scottish reorganisation process. Client access is described without emphasising the more simplified administrative structure of social work departments as compared with the two agencies of social services and probation departments. Again I am not criticising this study but only pointing to the way in which the author handles the material, apparently minimising the comparative differences.

A fourth reaction to the comparative problem is to *cope* with it. The objective of this strategy is to be in a position to make statements, of policy or professional significance, about social work and juvenile justice, which are applicable to Britain as a whole. The approach here is therefore to design a study in the context of one region and then simply to extend the sample to include a wider range of clients, social workers, agencies or whatever in order to support conclusions which are valid nationally. Comparative differences are not a part of the underlying logic of the research design and so these differences seldom feature systematically in the final report.

One example of this type of research is Stevenson *et al.* which is one of the few pieces of research in this field based upon English and Scottish (and Northern Irish) material.[42] The sample of 'social services departments and their equivalents in Scotland and Northern Ireland' included an English county and borough, two Scottish regions, two Northern Ireland boards, a Welsh county and a London borough. The objectives of the research are described as follows:

> our intention was to provide a detailed analysis of what social workers (and others relevant to their task) said they did, what they felt about their work and the organisation in which their work took place.

And the report notes:

> Social work in Scotland and Northern Ireland has special characteristics which the research team was bound to consider. Any account of this research which pretended that these, and other 'external' and organisational sources of difference did not exist would be sadly deficient.[43]

But because the study is not concerned to explain *why* social workers described their work in the way that they did no systematic attention is given to the impact upon those perceptions of variations along legal and organisational dimensions as between north and south Britain.[44] For example, in a chapter on 'specialisation' no particular feature is made of the separation of probation in the South. The main purpose throughout is to locate features of social workers' perceptions of social work which hold true for all areas, and thus advance national generalisations. There is therefore a tendency to identify a response arising with a particular context, not as a response *to* that context, but rather as an exemplification of a tendency of greater scope. The aim was to see that, so far as possible, 'all features of the contemporary scene were adequately covered'. That is consistent with the objectives which the research team set themselves. What is interesting in the light of the present discussion is that in spite of the fact that the project went to considerable trouble to collect data throughout Britain[45] the organisational and legal differences were not viewed as a major resource either in the design or analysis of the research.

And that is the main point that I am seeking to make in this section of the paper. Generally, it seems, social scientists view comparative differences in juvenile justice and social work systems within Britain as 'a trouble' in their work. The reactions to these differences which I have mentioned – ignore them, dismiss them, minimise them, cope with them – are reactions to a *problem*, and the strategies adopted are strategies for overcoming a hazard or an obstacle. An entirely different approach would be to view comparative differences as opportune rather than problematical, and as a rich resource to be exploited rather than as a snare to be evaded. In the next section I shall suggest how comparative policy research within Britain on juvenile justice and social work may adopt that stance.

Comparative differences as an opportunity

It is being argued in this paper that policy research should seek actively to capitalise upon the fact that social work, juvenile justice, and their interrelationship are conceptualised and organised in different ways within Britain. The paper is mainly about research relevant to social policies. Of course not all research on social work and juvenile justice is conducted with a major policy interest but some of the general arguments in the paper are applicable to investigations with more theoretical or methodological starting points too. The heart of the matter is that whatever the prime purpose of the investigation, we should question the apparent presumption that by extending data collection to areas north and south of the border the research task is *necessarily* complicated. Equally it may well be simplified. For research designs and data sources become available which might otherwise be excluded.

Indeed there is no very great difficulty in drawing up a list of topics which have featured recently in discussions of social work and delinquency and in then pointing to pertinent differences in the arrangements north and south of the border that might well afford opportunities for policy relevant research. For example, variations between juvenile courts and children's panels might be exploited to study variations in the perceptions of children and parents of 'welfare' as compared with 'judicial' systems of juvenile justice. It is a remarkable comment, both upon the parochial interests of social scientists and upon the initiative of research funding bodies, that a decade after major reforms both north and south of the border, there exists no sound basis for comparative experience in this field. To take another example, the varying patterns of responsibility between the Scottish Office on the one hand, and the Home Office and Department of Health and Social Security on the other, might be used to examine the effect of such arrangements upon policy issues. Studies of the different organisation of the probation service north and south of the border might shed much light on the issues of the so-called 'freedom' of southern probation from local authority control on the nature of 'specialist' as opposed to 'generic' social work, and on relation between social work and the judiciary under differing organisational arrangements. Variations between social work and social services departments might be studied to answer a whole host of questions about the relationship between patterns of administration and standards of service provision. Of course the conceptualisation of these questions demands refinement prior to data collection and analysis. There are no doubt other equally suitable topics and perhaps those topics which I have mentioned could also be researched in other ways. But that is not the point. All that I am intending to do here is to illustrate the argument that it is not unreasonable to presume *a priori* that comparative research will be useful and that in the area of social work and juvenile justice, data collection confined to either north or south Britain should be the exception rather than the rule.

Before leaving this point let me develop a little further, one more illustration of the way in which comparative differences in service provision may be viewed as an opportunity rather than as an obstacle to research. Shortly after the publication of the Seebohm report, and its reluctant confession that the committee's proposals were not based upon as much original research as would have been desirable, there followed a number of suggestions about how this deficiency could be rectified.[46] However, there was a major methodological difficulty in this field of research since the most obvious strategy was to call for data collection at two points in time in order to compare the operation of the social work system before and after the initiation of legislative and administrative change. Such research is seldom possible because policy initiatives are rarely announced with sufficient notice for the 'before' phase of data collection to be completed prior to the change and because retrospective data tends to be unreliable. That was certainly the case on this occasion and in consequence we have now no sound basis for comparing the performance of social work and social services departments, in relation to the services previously provided by the separate Children's, Welfare and other agencies.

Yet looking back at the issues which were seen as important at that time it is apparent that many of the central policy questions have not basically altered. Resources and public expenditure, the number of trained staff, the grounds of decision-making, reactions to social change, relations with other professions and agencies, client control, the 'bureaucratisation' of social work, client access, the categorisation of clients, and the role of volunteers – all retain significance. For these issues are at the heart of the service. Moreover, it is also apparent that the methodological problems of comparison over time may be surmounted by comparing instead the different systems which resulted from the re-organisation of social work and juvenile justice north and south of the border. So we have here a good example of precisely the general point that I am making. That is, differences in systems for the delivery of personal social services and juvenile justice in Britain may offer distinct advantages for policy research purposes and 'comparative' research across the differences is one way to exploit these advantages. As an extended illustration of the point, therefore, the following programme is offered to guide the collection of comparative material on the structure of juvenile justice and social work systems within Britain. The programme takes the form of a list of broad questions for research.

1. Do the different systems for delivering the personal social services and juvenile justice vary in the levels of public expenditure on these services? Are any variations related to the structure of service provision and what are their effects?

2. Are the different systems accompanied by variations in the use of trained staff? If so how are these variations to be explained and what are the consequences?

3. Do the different systems generate and use similar bodies of information for 'management' decision-taking and for making decisions about individual cases? If decisions are made on the basis of different material what are the causes and consequences of the differences?

4. Do the different systems evidence different reactions to the social changes in their environments and can any variation be related to organisational differences?

5. Do the different systems vary in the level of conflict, both experienced and witnessed, between social workers and other professional groups – for example, teachers, nurses, administrators, doctors, the judiciary and the police? How are these differences to be explained?

6. Do the different systems vary in the level of conflict, both experienced and witnessed, between the departments of personal social services and local authority departments such as health, housing and education?

7. Are variations apparent between the different systems in the part that clients and social workers play in the control of service provision? If so, are variations related to the organisation of the services?

8. Are different patterns of 'bureaucratisation' apparent between the systems and if so how does this influence service delivery?

9. Are the social services offered within the two systems used by

different cross sections of the population and do the different systems have a different effect upon client access to the services?

10. Do the different systems vary in the conceptual models, and categories of service provision, which service providers employ to classify the problems and needs of clients and their own particular skills? Are any variations related to the administrative framework of the services?

11. How does the use of volunteers vary between the systems and what are the results of these differences?

12. What major differences in the personal social services of the two systems follow from the retention of a separate administration for the probation service in the south?

The real problem of the differences

Up to now in this paper I have been arguing that differences in systems of personal social service and juvenile justice in Britain present no major problem for research. On the contrary, they represent an opportunity. However, having made this point, it is difficult to avoid the sensation that it is really rather obvious and unexceptionable. Indeed it seems odd that it is necessary to make the point at all. Yet the paucity of existing research, and also the way in which the whole topic is glossed over in the literature, indicate clearly that it is. The question therefore arises as to why, in the face of its promise and advantages, comparative research within Britain on social work and related services should have been so neglected and, indeed, one feels positively discouraged by the predominant trends in policy studies. Suggestions about future research programmes may be interesting but they do little to remove the doubt that if comparative research on social welfare has been hitherto so unpopular there is no clear reason why that situation should now change.

One response might be that the substantive advantages of comparative research are clear but the theoretical and methodological problems are formidable. Certainly there are complications in comparative methodology and research on the personal social services and juvenile justice escapes them no more easily than research in other areas of social policy. There is the problem that I have already mentioned that variation in so many factors makes it difficult to control for limited differences. Comparative studies must also avoid the somewhat atheoretical approach which characterises much of the so-called descriptive research in social welfare. There are major methodological problems in the comparative use of official statistics and problems of standardising the methods of data collection for other kinds of material as well.

There is also one theoretical problem which is particularly pertinent to the area of research discussed here. So far in this paper I have used the notion of 'legal and administrative structure' (or some such term) and have suggested that this should be the initial focus for research because of the paucity of material on other aspects of the services, especially in social work. But I have used the notion rather loosely and as soon as we begin to study a service in any detail this gives rise to difficulty. First, it is typically a matter of dispute as to what constitutes the basis of the formal structure. For example, guidelines on the use of section 12 produced by a director of social work and distributed in mimeographed form and on a confidential basis within the department might be viewed as binding by fieldworkers, advisory by the social work committee and a component of the department's informal discretion by central government. In fact what 'is' and 'is not' agency structure may well be employed as a resource to either validate or discredit components of the organisation in which different groups have vested interests. Thus whether they realise it or not social scientists describing the structure of an agency soon begin to take sides in political disputes.[47]

The second difficulty is that rules require interpretation. It is extremely hard to get any picture of a strange service simply by studying legislation or even supplementary regulations. In the absence of further data social scientists are inclined to fill the gaps with anecdotal and impressionistic material, often in unspecified ways. The literature on the children's panels is replete with descriptions of the system which purport to be straightforward accounts of the legal and administrative structure but which necessarily invoke much interpretation of what particular rules and policies mean. For the structure of a service is interpreted and takes shape through the concepts, ideologies and routine practices of professionals, administrators, clerical staff, laymen and clients who interact through the business of service provision. So there is a problem in supposing that 'legal and administrative structure', on the one hand, and 'professional practice' or 'service delivery', on the other, may be conceptualised and measured as separate variables. Yet many of the research questions that I have posed in this paper call, basically, for measures of service provision between systems in the light of the known (measured) variations in the legal and administrative structure.

Nevertheless, theoretical and methodological difficulties are far from unknown in any type of social policy research and in spite of the problems that I have mentioned it is hard to see that comparative studies are distinctive in this respect. As I have already mentioned, all research is in a sense 'comparative' and in any case it is hard to see why contrasts *within* Britain should not be made when contrasts *between* Britain and other nation states frequently are. It is also true that many other kinds of research proceed more or less satisfactorily, in spite of widely acknowledged but still unsolved methodological difficulties. For example, although the literature on 'qualitative methods' is relatively sophisticated, in practice the collection of data gathering activities which are grouped under the umbrella category of 'participant observation' render the validation or replication of many studies quite impossible. Yet this approach is still adopted in much social work research. To give another example, the unreliable nature of official statistics is well known and much debated, as I have already mentioned, yet a major part of delinquency research continues, simply by ignoring the point. The difficulties in effective evaluation are massive yet this remains the stock in trade of social policy studies. It is widely argued that the model of a clinical trial is inappropriate to social work yet such designs are still attempted, and successful projects are quoted as examples of sophisticated research. It is known that there is a problematic relationship between descriptions of their behaviour given by professionals and clients in interview and their observed practices, yet both interviews and questionnaires are extensively used with scant regard to this relationship. Research, at least in social work and juvenile justice, is no different from any other social institution in failing to live up to the standards of its own utopian ideals,[48] while nevertheless continuing to function successfully according to alternative criteria. An explanation for the paucity of comparative research in this field cannot therefore rest solely in its theoretical and methodological complexities. A full account must lie elsewhere.

In concluding this paper then I want to suggest that institutional rather than intellectual factors have inhibited the intra-Britain comparative study of systems for delivering juvenile justice and the personal social services. These very brief comments are made with a view to considering what action may be required to promote this type of research in the future, and it may be useful to place discussion under the five headings of funding, staffing, managing, publishing and implementing research. The general point that I am hypothesising is that research problems like all social problems, are socially situated in a specific organisational and political context, and it is thus the structure of welfare research itself which has rendered it incapable of either generating, sustaining or investigating the significant comparative questions in this field.

As so often in social policy, the first thing to consider is finance. There seems no particular reason why funding from research council or trust fund sources should have inhibited comparative studies, but much of the research on juvenile justice and the personal social services is supported from government funds. The most relevant sources are the Home Office, Department of Health and Social Security, Scottish Home and Health Department and the Social Work Services Group. Since research votes are tied to departments and used in alliance with departmental interests, and since comparative research by its very nature crosses and even endangers these interests, it is not an area to which any substantial funds have been assigned. Joint funding is not a practice which finds favour in central government. Local government supports very little external research and its interests are, in any case, parochial. The resources of bodies such as CCETSW or the PSSC which might have had more active interests in comparative studies have been limited too. Comparative research also tends to be rather expensive because of the amount of travel involved, the need to duplicate secretarial and clerical support and the general costs of coordinated activity.

A second most important resource for comparative research is personnel. The problem of competence has already been mentioned and although this may not be *so* important in a context confined to Britain, there have been relatively few research staff available with prior research experience both north and south of the border. The staffing position in universities may well reduce geographical mobility in the immediate future and this is significant if it is true that comparative research tends to arise, initially, at the suggestion of individuals who have a personal interest in both areas. Within central government research staff tend not to move around between departments in the way that is frequent amongst senior administrators.

However, the most formidable organisational problems of comparative research may well arise in the actual management of the project. Since, in practice, most research changes as it progresses, however rigorous the initial design, there are always problems of coordinating intellectual perspectives and practical activities within a research team. Combined with the logistic problems of data collection in separate sites these hazards may be particularly formidable in comparative research. One way of overcoming such problems is to work with a team of researchers who have shared a common perspective over a period of time. However, because of the structure of research, units of this kind, although they are not unknown, are the exception rather than the rule. The permanent research units investigating social work and juvenile justice in central government are located within particular departments and, for the reasons that I have already mentioned are not, apparently, inclined to undertake programmes of comparative research.

Finally, the hurdles of publication and especially implementation appear daunting for comparative studies within Britain. Certainly many authors gain the impression that it is crucial to be able to demonstrate to publishers a rather direct and clear relevance to the English market. Insufficient attention has been paid to the relationship between the financial and marketing aspects of publishing (both books and journals) and the directions taken by social science research. But it seems likely that this relationship accounts for the strategy of 'minimising the problem of the differences' which I discussed earlier.

Likewise most policy researchers will look for some identifiable 'consumer' for their work with a view (however unrealistic) to implementation. But by its very nature comparative research may have no obvious 'customer' and implementation may be particularly complex. Learning practical lessons from comparative research is never easy. One suspects that it is particularly difficult if the lesson is to be learned close to home. To put the point perhaps somewhat crudely, there may be no easier way of ensuring that a government department does not change its policies, than by announcing that you have discovered that the 'Auld Enemy' has found a way of doing it better.

Conclusion

I have concluded this paper with some slightly speculative comments geared to explaining the paucity of comparative research on varying systems within Britain for the delivery of personal social service and juvenile justice. These comments have reflected the view that studies in social policy are reflexive. They arise out of the stuff which is the object of their investigations. That is, we do not need what Blume calls the unnecessary simplying assumption that (social) science is an autonomous sub-system insulated from social, economic and political dynamics in society.[49] As Crawford and Perry note in introducing *Demands for Social Knowledge*, 'research activity is shaped by demands for knowledge by social agents other than disciplinary peers'.[50]

Thus any completely adequate statement about the condition of comparative studies in this field requires a much broader analysis than I have been able to offer in this paper. But in these notes I have tried to make a start by suggesting that if we agree, as I have supposed, that the organisational structure of service delivery in social work and juvenile justice has an effect on service delivery, then it is equally reasonable to suppose that the organisation of research in this field has an impact upon the prevalence of comparative studies.

Of course that does not release us from the obligation to spell out a programme of comparative research, and I have sought to illustrate the way in which that should proceed. I have pointed to the most obvious differences between the systems in north and south Britain, described the most usual reactions to these differences in the literature and made some suggestions which at least indicate that comparative research is likely to be fruitful. In pointing to some of the proposals for research which follow the recommendations of the Seehohm report I offered, in particular, an example of the way in which comparative research within Britain could be exploited to overcome the difficulties of evaluative research over time.

Naturally there are theoretical and methodological complications but this particular type of research is far from unique in that respect. The explanation for the paucity of comparative research must lie elsewhere. It seems naive, therefore, to advocate such a programme of research without also considering why this approach has not been actively pursued before. The answer apparently lies more in the way in which research is funded, staffed, managed, published and implemented, than in its intrinsic merits. For certainly the way in which the reogranisation of social work and juvenile justice has taken place in Britain would seem to have made this area of policy, perhaps above all others, ideally suited to the constructive use of comparative experience.

Notes

1. This article is a revised version of a paper commissioned by the SSRC and originally presented at the Workshop on the Comparative Study of the Social Services in the United Kingdom and Eire, University of Edinburgh, September 1979.
2. 'The personal social services' is a term which is used here to refer to what is often simply called 'social work'. See R. A. Pinker, *Research Priorities in the Personal Social Services, London*: Social Science Research Council, 1978, and Eric Sainsbury, *The Personal Social Services*, London: Pitman, 1977. The term tends to be employed in order to avoid the objections of social workers who may argue that this latter function is a more specialised and skilled activity capable of being performed only be trained and professionally qualified staff. This narrower view would exclude, for example, the work of the home help service. It is sometimes argued that Social Work Departments in Scotland are misnamed since these agencies do much else besides social work, and that, in spite of their more limited functions, Social Services Departments are more accurately titled.

   'Juvenile justice' is a term which has gained some currency since the publication of Aaron V. Cicourel's *The Social Organisation of Juvenile Justice*, New York: Wiley, 1968, and describes the network of a variety of agencies that form the system for dealing with delinquent children or those in need of care where some measure of compulsion is employed. Some agencies in this system take decisions. Some offer treatment programmes and vary from prisons to social work agencies.
3. In the context of the Workshop in which this paper was originally presented, the exclusion of Northern Ireland was hard to defend.
4. This whole area of research is a veritable minefield of terminological dangers. It is symptomatic of the political features of comparative research that there is dispute about the exact scope of 'Britain', 'Great Britain', and the 'United Kingdom'. The Oxford Dictionary defines 'Britain' as 'The proper name of the whole island containing England, Wales and Scotland, with their dependencies; more fully called Great Britain; now used for the British empire as a whole'; 'United Kingdom' as, 'the kingdom of Great Britain or (from 1801 to 1922) of Great Britain and Ireland'; and 'England' as 'The southern part of the island of

Great Britain. Occas. loosely: Great Britain. Often: The English (or British) nation or state'. Neither 'Ireland' nor 'Eire' is listed, but 'Irish Free State' is 'the part of Ireland separated from the U.K. and established as a Dominion 1922'. 'Scotland' appears only as 'Scotland Yard'. In this article I shall use 'Britain' to mean England, Wales and Scotland, and I shall be comparing Scotland with England and Wales.

5. There is now a ready source of reference to the distinctive features of the welfare state in Scotland in J. English and F. M. Martin (eds.), *Social Services in Scotland*, Edinburgh: Scottish Academic Press, 1979.
6. Some of these points are developed more fully in Gilbert Smith, *Social Need; Policy, Practice, and Research*, London and Boston: Routledge and Kegan Paul, 1980.
7. The major official publications relevant here are (in date order): *Report of the Committee on Children and Young Persons* (The Ingleby Report), Cmnd 1191, London: HMSO, 1960; Children and Young Persons Act, London: HMSO, 1963; *Prevention and Neglect of Children*, (The McBoyle Report), Cmnd 1966, Edinburgh: HMSO, 1963; *Children and Young Persons, Scotland* (The Kilbrandon Report), Cmnd 2306, Edinburgh: HMSO, 1964; *The Child, The Family and the Young Offender*, Cmnd 2742, London: HMSO, 1965; *Social Work and the Community*, Cmnd 3065, Edinburgh: HMSO, 1966; *Children in Trouble*, Cmnd 3601, London: HMSO, 1968; *Report of the Committee on Local Authority and Allied Personal Social Services* (The Seebohm Report), Cmnd 3703, London: HMSO, 1968; Social Work (Scotland) Act, London: HMSO, 1968; *Children and Young Persons Act*, London: HMSO, 1969; *Local Authority Social Services Act*, London: HMSO, 1970.
8. See Jean Packman, *The Child's Generation: Child Care Policy from Curtis to Houghton*, Oxford and London: Basil Blackwell and Martin Robertson, 1975.
9. Phoebe Hall, *Reforming the Welfare: The Politics of Change in the Personal Social Services*, London: Heinemann, 1976.
10. There are notable exceptions. See: E. M. Goldberg and D. J. Fruin, 'Towards Accountability in Social Work: A Case Review System for Social Workers', *British Journal of Social Work*, Vol. 6, 1976, pp. 3–22; E. M. Goldberg *et al.*, 'Towards Accountability in Social Work. One Year's Intake to an Area Office', *British Journal of Social Work*, Vol. 7, 1977, pp. 257–83; E. M. Goldberg *et al.*, 'Towards Accountability in Social Work: Long Term Social Work in an Area Office', *British Journal of Social Work*, Vol. 8, 1978, pp. 253–87; Olive Stevenson *et al.*, *Social Service Teams: The Practitioner's View*, London: HMSO. Also most local authorities have established small research teams within their social services departments and the work from these units is brought together by a clearing house based at the University of Birmingham. However much of this work takes the form of local intelligence, and it is hard to draw any theoretically informed general conclusions. Eric Sainsbury's much quoted study, *Social Work with Families*, London and Boston: Routledge and Kegan Paul, 1975, draws data from Family Service Units.
11. *Report of the Committee on Local Authority and Allied Personal Social Services.*
12. See note 7 for a full list of the relevant official publications.
13. The juvenile court in Scotland prior to the creation of the Children's panel system was a Sheriff court with the exception of four local authority areas which possessed a specially constituted Justice of the Peace (Juvenile) Court on an experimental basis under the provisions of the 1937 Children and Young Persons (Scotland) Act. These JP (Juvenile) Courts resembled the Juvenile Courts in England and Wales. So far as I am aware there is no systematic research comparison of these institutions and those of the more usual pattern informed the decision to establish Children's Panels. This is another example of the point that sufficient variation may well be available within regions to facilitate research.

14. Social Work (Scotland) Act 1968, S.12 (1) and (4).
15. *Reforming the Welfare: The Politics of Change in the Personal Social Services.*
16. Stuart Rees, *Social Work Face to Face*, London: Edward Arnold, 1978.
17. Margaret Voysey, *A Constant Burden: The Reconstitution of Family Life*, London and Boston: Routledge and Kegan Paul, 1975.
18. Mildred Blaxter, *The Meaning of Disability*, London: Heinemann, 1976.
19. *Social Service Teams: The Practitioner's View.*
20. M. P. Jackson and B. M. Valencia, *Financial Aid Through Social Work*, London and Boston: Routledge and Kegan Paul, 1979.
21. J. H. Curran, *The Children's Hearing System: A Review of Research*, Edinburgh: HMSO, 1977.
22. See, for example, David May, 'The Children's Hearing System. Part 1. The Limits to Legislative Action', *Journal of Social Welfare Law*, Vol. 1, pp. 14–23, 1978.
23. Nigel Bruce and John Spencer, *Face to Face with Families*, Loanhead Midlothian: Macdonald publishers, 1976.
24. A. Morris with M. MacIsacc, *Juvenile Justice?* London: Heinemann, 1978.
25. F. M. Martin, S. Fox and K. Murray, *Children Out of Court*, Edinburgh: Scottish Academic Press, 1981.
26. F. M. Martin, and K. Murray (eds.), *Children's Hearings*, Edinburgh: Scottish Academic Press, 1976.
27. P. D. Brown and T. Bloomfield (eds.), *Legality and Community: The Politics of Juvenile Justice in Scotland*, Aberdeen: People's Press, 1979.
28. Phylida Parsloe, *Juvenile Justice in Britain and the United States*, London and Boston; Routledge and Kegan Paul, 1978.
29. As also with those articles on Scottish juvenile justice which are to be found in international comparative volumes. See Beti Jones and G. J. Murray, 'The Scottish Rejection of the Juvenile Court', Chapter 6 in V. Lorne Stewart (ed.), *The Changing Face of Juvenile Justice*, New York: University Press, 1978; and J. C. Spencer, 'Children's Hearings in Scotland', pp. 257–72, in I. F. G. Baxter and M. A. Eberts (eds.), *The Child and the Courts*, Toronto: Carswell, London: Sweet and Maxwell, 1978.
30. I have not mentioned the possible use of official statistics as a basis for comparative research. The methodological debate on this topic, particularly in relation to delinquency statistics, has raged in the literature from J. I. Kitsuse and A. V. Cicourel's, 'A Note on the Use of Official Statistics' (*Social Problems*, Vol. 11, 1963, pp. 131–9) onwards. In outline the problems are that (i) one cannot be sure whether the structure or performance of a system is being measured; (ii) the purposes and interests of the parties generating the data need to be understood; and (iii) there is a circular process in which, 'Their [record-makers] investigative procedures are rooted in particular conceptions of the social world and these conceptions are then reinforced by the results of such investigative procedures.' (Sally Macintyre, 'Some Notes on Record Taking and Making in an Antenatal Clinic', *The Sociological Review*, Vol. 26, 1978, pp. 595–611). Most recently, see John Irvine *et al.* (eds.), *Demystifying Social Statistics*, London: Pluto Press, 1977; and Sally Macintyre's constructive note on how empirical investigations may facilitate the use of official records and statistics as resources for social scientific research. Any major research programme on this theme would take up these points, but they are beyond the immediate scope of this article.
31. Some but not all, courses in Scotland are recognised by the Home Office as equipping students to practise as probation officers in the South. Some Scottish courses may contain options on, say, 'work with offenders', amongst other options but this leads to no distinctive qualification.
32. Chapter 3 in R. G. S. Brown's, *The Management of Welfare* (Glasgow: Fontana/Collins, 1975) is a model of exposition on the structure of central government but is confined to the DHSS. A ready source of comparative data on the way

in which central government classifies and groups its responsibilities is available in the 'Distribution of Business' handbook for each department, unfortunately generally marked, 'NOT TO BE DISCLOSED TO ANYONE OUTSIDE THE PUBLIC SERVICE'.

33. But see English and Martin, *Social Services in Scotland.*
34. T. H. Marshall, *Social Policy*, (new edn.), London: Hutchinson, 1975.
35. Muriel Brown, *Introduction to Social Administration in Britain* (3rd edn.), London: Hutchinson, 1976.
36. David C. Marsh (ed.), *Introducing Social Policy*, London and Boston: Routledge and Kegan Paul, 1979, p. ix.
37. Eric Sainsbury, *The Personal Social Services*, London: Pitman, 1977.
38. *Financial Aid Through Social Work*.
39. *Financial Aid Through Social Work*. p. 3.
40. *Financial Aid Through Social Work*. p. 3.
41. *Social Work Face to Face*.
42. *Social Service Teams: The Practitioner's View*.
43. *Social Service Teams: The Practitioner's View*, pp. 10, 11.
44. This is not to say that comparisons are never made. For instance differences in referral patterns of mental health work to area teams are noted and an explanation is offered in terms of the difference between section 29 of the Mental Health Act 1959 and section 31 of the Mental Health (Scotland) Act 1960 (pp. 36–77).
45. The research was financed by grants from the Department of Health and Social Security, the Department of Health and Social Services (Northern Ireland) and the Social Work Services Group of the Scottish Education Department. It entailed two research teams: one based at Aberdeen and the other at Oxford and Keele.
46. Some of these suggestions were set out in a paper commissioned by the SSRC. See *SSRC Newsletter*, Vol. 10, November 1970 and Gilbert Smith, 'Some Research Implications of the Seebohm Report', *British Journal of Sociology*, Vol. XXII, pp. 295–310, 1971.
47. See Howard S. Becker's classic statement of this dilemma in research, 'Whose Side Are We On?', *Social Problems*, Vol. 44, 1967, pp. 239–47.
48. See Colin Bell and Howard Newby, *Doing Sociological Research*, London: George Allen and Unwin, 1977.
49. Stewart S. Blume, *Towards a Political Sociology of Science*, New York: Free Press, 1974.
50. Elizabeth Crawford and Norman Perry (eds.), *Demands for Social Knowledge*, London and Beverly Hills, California: Sage, 1976, p. 9.

8 Northern Ireland's Integrated Health and Personal Social Service Structure

Derek Birrell and *Arthur Williamson*

The reorganisation of health and personal social services in Northern Ireland in 1973 stemmed from two basic factors – a desire to follow proposals for the reorganisation of the National Health Service in Great Britain and a decision to reform local government in Northern Ireland. Eventually the reorganisation was to become part of a much larger reorganisation of local administration brought about as a response to the demands for social and political reforms in the late 1960s.

Northern Ireland has had a system of integrated welfare departments since 1948, when eight welfare authorities for the six County Councils and two County Boroughs were established. The health service was organised on lines similar to Britain through a central Northern Ireland Hospitals Authority, a General Health Services Board, and eight local authority health committees.

A Social Services financial agreement[1] in 1949 between the Northern Ireland and Westminster governments required the Northern Ireland Government to maintain the scale and standard of comprehensive health services in Northern Ireland in general conformity with the scale and standard of such services in Great Britain. This did not rule out opportunities for experimentation or differences in the administrative structure of services. For example Northern Ireland developed a Special Care Service providing what today would be called a 'programme of care' approach for the mentally handicapped under which medical, residential, occupational, educational and social work care was coordinated. A further example was the integration of hospital and community provision for patients suffering from tuberculosis which was coordinated through the Northern Ireland Tuberculosis Authority. Personal social services were also mainly kept in parity with Great Britain although here again there were some significant differences. For example in 1968 Northern Ireland introduced a Children and Young Persons Act which was essentially similar to the 1963 Act in Great Britain. But Northern Ireland has not yet introduced legislation similar to the 1969 Children and Young Persons Act in Britain. Legislation on adoption was different until 1966 when Northern Ireland had to amend its legislation to enable the United Kingdom to sign the 1965 Hague Convention on adoption.

In the late 1960s the Northern Ireland Government produced two papers with proposals for the reform of the existing local government structure.[2]

Table 8.1 Local government structure pre 1973

County Boroughs	2	County Councils	6
		Borough Councils	10
		Urban Districts	24
		Rural Districts	31

The second of these documents, published in July 1969, proposed a single tier system of seventeen authorities and raised a question about the future administration of social services by the county councils. It noted that the Northern Ireland Government had decided to invite discussion of an integration of the three sectors of the health services along lines similar to Great Britain and also concerning a new structure for personal social services and education. Shortly afterwards the Government published a Green Paper, *The Administrative Structure of the Health and Personal Social Services in Northern Ireland.*[3] This paper proposed the integration of the three parts of the health service under a system of nominated Area Boards, largely along lines similar to the equivalent British proposals. The reasons given for this change were also similar to those in the 1968 English Green Paper; that the existing structure was tripartite while the individual's needs should be seen as a continuum; that the separate branches of the health services were becoming increasingly independent in treatment and care, and that a single authority for each area could more easily secure the most effective use of available resources.[4] The Green Paper rejected the possibility of a single health board for Northern Ireland referring to the problems which would arise from depriving local interests of an adequate say in determining local provision.

If the proposals on the reorganisation of health services followed the mainland example, the thinking of the Green Paper on the personal social services did not. The Green Paper proposed the integration of health and personal social services under an area board structure. The decision to integrate health and social services received remarkably little discussion in the Green Paper apart from a few references to 'the need for cooperation and joint planning becoming increasingly recognised', and assertions that 'the best framework for the continued development of personal social services is to be found in their coming into some form of parternship with health services'. The main reasons discussed in the Green Paper referred mainly to administrative factors. Separate social work departments would have increased the number of administrative bodies and the number of administrative staff and supporting resources and would have made coordination between social work and the health services more difficult.

After a series of consultations and meetings with the interests concerned the Government was able to state that there was widespread support for the principle of integration of the administrative structure of the health services and 'considerable acceptance' of the concept of a single set of Boards administering health and personal social services together with safeguards to preserve the separate identity of the personal social services.

The Green Paper proposals were closely linked in timing and substance with the reorganisation of local government. While the consultations on the Green Paper were being completed the Government appointed a Review Body on Local Government and a final decision on health and personal social services had to await its findings. The Review Body's *Report* (The Macrory Report)[5] in July 1970 largely endorsed the Green Paper Proposals. In December 1970 the Government announced its intentions of replacing the existing local government structure with a single tier of twenty-six district councils while the major public and social services would be centralised. Personal health and personal social services would become regional responsibilities of the Department of Health and Social Services and would be administered through an Area Board structure.

In 1971 a Consultative Document[6] was published with the detailed proposals for the new structure and was shortly followed by the legislative proposals. The proposed restructuring received a rather cautious welcome from the social work profession. There was little objection to the removal of personal social services from local councils. Concern was expressed that the final proposals fell short of the concept of unified personal social services, even as outlined in the Green Paper, by excluding community work, educational welfare, child guidance and probation. There was also some apprehension about integration with the National Health Service. It was felt that the greatly imbalanced division of resources as between health and social services would seriously weaken the notion of corporate management. Social workers were generally rather apprehensive about the likely effectiveness of separate social work committees and directors as a guarantee against domination by the health service and the medical profession.

Medical opinion was largely in favour of the proposals but the decision to have four boards ran counter to the advice of the powerful medical lobby which wanted a single statutory body to administer all the health and personal social services in the region. This line of argument was resisted by government on the grounds that while planning could be centralised, management could not; that the DHSS(NI) already was performing the functions of a body such as was suggested; and that the most successful administrative arrangement would comprise one level – Government – responsible for strategic planning and resource allocation, and a number of second tier bodies charged with the management, operational planning, and delivery of services.

Expected advantages

The new structure held promise of a number of important benefits for the people of Northern Ireland and for the staff working within it. The Permanent Secretary of DHSS(NI), speaking in May 1971, identified the main advantages of the new system in the following terms. It would make comprehensive planning possible at every level and would encompass the totality of medical and social care. It would make possible a more rational grouping of professional resources and facilities. It would remove the archaic structure of forty-seven bodies which were providers of medical and social care. These would be replaced with four Area Boards which would much more easily identify with their geographical areas and the populations for which they would become responsible. Public participation was to be assured at both levels: at Board level by the participation of community representatives; at district level by district committees.[7]

Reorganisation was, therefore, an attempt to achieve a wide range of objectives. It would bring together into a rational framework services which had grown in isolation and would provide channels of communication and cooperation between different groups of caring professionals. Integration and coordination would increase, it was argued, as understanding grew between the professions and as priorities were agreed on the basis of identified medical and social need rather than conflicting professional perspectives. The identification of main patient/client groups such as the elderly and the physically and mentally handicapped was an attempt to put the needs of patients and clients before the interests of professions existing to meet those needs.

The establishment of four boards with their headquarters in leading provincial towns would also, it was hoped, demagnetise Belfast and, consistent with regional physical development strategy, would provide a series of major centres which would balance Belfast's almost inexorable tendency to dominate the province and to consume an inordinate proportion of the resources of the services.

Implementation

The process of reorganisation took place in a remarkably smooth manner between 1971 and 1973 despite the surrounding political turmoil and civil disturbances. The legislation bringing in the new system eventually passed through the Westminster Parliament as an Order-in-Council following the suspension of the Stormont Parliament in March 1972. A team of management consultants[8] was engaged to advise on the planning and management of the structure and worked as part of a project team with officers from the services and with a steering group from the Department. The recommendations of the project team and steering group were the basis for the reorganised structure which came into operation in October 1973.

The new structure for the services in Northern Ireland had been developed by a civil service responsible to the Stormont Parliament. But that Parliament had disappeared in March 1972 and with it the Cabinet, local ministerial control and, most important, a provincial forum for policy-making and responsive political interaction. The civil disturbances also made Northern Ireland an unattractive place to which to try to recruit staff to man the higher echelons of the professional and administrative structure. This was to prove a particularly intractable problem in the case of the medical administration and was accentuated by the opportunities created by the reorganisation of the National Health Service in Britain at the same time.

The Department of Health and Social Services has the duty of providing health and personal social services, decides overall policy, priorities and standards, finances the services and supervises the capital works programme. The Department delegates to four Area Boards the planning and delivery of services within their respective areas. Members of the Area Boards are appointed by the Minister. About 30% represent the professions, a further 30% are nominated by local government District Councils and the remainder represent industry, trade unions, universities and voluntary bodies. The total membership of the boards ranges from 24 to 33. Each board has a number of statutory committees. These are a Health Services Committee, a Policy and Resources Committee, a Personal Social Services Committee and an Administrative Services Committee. The chief officers of each board include a Chief Administrative Officer, a Chief Administrative Medical Officer, a Chief Administrative Nursing Officer and a Director of Social Services. Together with the Chairman of the Area Medical Advisory Committee they form the Executive Team.

Each area comprises and is conterminous with a number of local government districts, and these districts, either singly or in groups, form district units for the local delivery of health and personal social services,

Prior to the 1982 reorganisation there were three such districts for the Belfast area and fourteen for the rest of the province. District officers corresponding to the area officers formed a District Executive Team. The area and district teams were intended to work on the basis of corporate management. In each of the districts there is a district committee which represents the interests of the consumer and the local community and acts in an advisory capacity. The district committee is appointed by the appropriate Area Board.

There were a number of activities which it was thought could best be organised on a regional basis outside rather than inside the Department. A Central Services Agency provides certain common services on behalf of the Department and the Boards. It makes payments to contractors like general practitioners, chemists and opticians, arranges for the selection and appointment of senior medical staff, provides legal services for the Boards and places central contracts for supplies. A Staffs Council for Health and Social Services develops common selection and appointment procedures and provides some personnel and training services. Certain clinical specialities, research activities and the Blood Transfusion Service are also organised on a regional basis and are administered by the Eastern Board.

In 1975 a Departmental Paper *Regional Strategy for the Development of Health and Personal Social Services in Northern Ireland*[9] saw the strategic aims and objectives of the health and personal social services as beginning to emerge clearly and definitively from the new structure. The overall objective was declared to be the promotion of high-quality and cost-effective services provided on a coordinated and accessible basis and delivered in a manner which is acceptable to individuals and communities. This paper noted the imbalance between care in the hospital and care in the community and that community health and social care were still comparatively underdeveloped. While noting increasing financial restraints the paper called for the development of community health and social care, particularly for the mentally handicapped, the mentally ill, the physically handicapped, the elderly and other priority categories, including children and young people at risk.

Evaluation of the 1973 reorganisation

After ten years it is possible to make some assessment of the operation of the integrated structure of health and personal social services. It is clear that serious problems began to emerge in the late 1970s in relation to the administrative structure, and this led the Government to produce proposals for some further restructuring. The Government was also strongly influenced by the publication of the Royal Commission's *Report on the National Health Service*[10] with its recommendations that it was necessary to review existing management structures, the professional advisory structure and ensure that local management was more effective. The Royal Commission had also suggested each health department in the different parts of the United Kingdom should initiate a review of the structure for which it was responsible. In 1979, the Department of Health and Social Services published a *Consultative Paper*[11] on the scope for improvement in the structure, organisation and management arrangements of the health and personal social services. The Department then established a Joint Review Group of officials to review the evidence gathered by the Department in consultation with the interests involved and to make recommendations on the way forward. A *Review*[12] of medical participation and advice in the management structure was also prepared by the Chief Medical Officer of the Department of Health and Social Services (Northern Ireland). In June 1981 the Government published its decisions on restructuring in a Departmental Circular.[13]

An assessment of the operation of the integrated structure is now made under six headings which identify the key problem areas: Department/regional matters, the administrative structure of areas and districts, medical advisory machinery, public participation and accountability, professional integration and the integration of social work with the health services. In examining these issues reference is made to the findings and recommendations contained in the document prepared by the Joint Review Group[14] and to the decisions announced in the Departmental Circular.[15]

Department, regional matters

In Northern Ireland, as in Scotland and Wales, there is no regional authority separate from the Department of Health and Social Services. The four Health and Social Service Boards relate directly to the Department. Since 1973 there has been considerable dissatisfaction among the Area Boards with the role of the Department. These criticisms relate mainly to the assertion that the Department was sometimes rigid and often unpredictable in the discharge of its coordination responsibilities, that it failed to delegate effectively and also involved itself in functions properly the responsibility of Boards.

A further focus of criticism related to the fact that civil service personnel have much less continuity of function than would be the case in a Regional Health Authority. This had, it was claimed, led to unnecessary frustration as relationships between senior Board and Department officers were continually fractured because of reshuffling of Department staff within the Civil Service structure. It was also claimed that civil servants rarely possessed the expertise in health and social service planning questions and the detailed knowledge and sensitivity which might be expected from the staff of a regional authority.

Other criticisms of the Department's regional role concerned poor communication within the Department, inadequacies in the machinery for planning regional medical and dental services and inadequacies in the regional support and advisory services provided to Boards by the Department's Research and Intelligence and Work's Units by the Central Services Agency and the Staffs Council. Undoubtedly some of the criticisms and alleged shortcomings were framed in the light of comparisons with the defunct Northern Ireland Hospitals' Authority which existed until replaced by the Area Boards in 1973 and which was much favoured by the medical profession.

As in 1972 the most insistent advocate of a regional authority was the British Medical Association, now joined by the British Dental Association. These bodies advocated the setting up of a regional authority which would exercise certain of the Department's resource allocation, regional planning and monitoring functions and would also take over the functions of the Central Services Agency and the Staffs Council. They also wished to see the creation of a parallel Central Contractor's Bureau at regional level which would be responsible for independent contractor services on a basis similar to Family Practitioner Committees in England. This would have replaced the arrangements whereby Health and Social Service Boards hold the contracts of all independent contractors.

These recommendations were rejected by the Advisory Group appointed by the Minister of State. It considered that the creation of a regional authority would ignore the existence of the area as a viable planning unit and that it would conflict with the principles of the new management arrangements in Great Britain recommending that the planning level should normally serve populations of between 150,000 and 500,000. Problems would also have arisen in the field of accountability; since a Regional Authority could not itself be accountable to Parliament and, since the Permanent Secretary is the Accounting Officer for the service with responsibility for the allocation and use of resources, continued departmental involvement would have been necessary, were there to be a Regional Authority. This would, it was argued, inevitably lead to undesirable duplication of, and confusion of, roles.

With regard to independent contractor services, the Advisory Group recommended that the setting up of such bodies would necessarily further distance general practitioners from Area Boards and would therefore inhibit integration of community services.

Areas, districts and units of management

One of the most persistent difficulties in operating the structure set up in 1973 was administrative overlap between the roles of areas and districts. These problems were experienced throughout Northern Ireland but most acutely in the North and West District of Belfast in which are located the Royal Group of Hospitals and which, during the 1970s, experienced levels of social deprivation and violence unique in the British Isles.[16] Management issues that were common across Northern Ireland were experienced there with unique intensity, reflecting both the peculiarly complex nature of the administrative problems of the district and its ever present backdrop of grave social need.

Following the 1973 reorganisation Area Executive Teams (AETs) were made up of a Chief Administrative Officer, a Chief Administrative Medical Officer, a Director of Social Services, a Chief Nursing Officer and a second medical representative of the Area medical advisory machinery. Chief Officers are responsible to their boards and had responsible to them, until the recent reorganisation, a number of DETs (District Executive Teams). Both AETs and DETs were expected to operate on a corporate basis and the area Chief Officers were responsible for the work of district officers in a line management sense.

It was unrealistic in 1973 to expect that sufficient numbers of appropriately trained and experienced officers would be found to fill over 120 senior professional posts in the area and district structure and it soon became obvious that the service was becoming overadministered and undermanaged. It is sometimes suggested that the roots of this weakness in the structure stemmed from the brief given to the management consultants who planned the district administrative structure. It is claimed that they planned the district level with insufficient information about its anticipated size and that the functions and structure of the area were decided after the district structure had been settled.

Seventeen districts were set up in 1973. This number, and the consequent small size of districts, was a response to what was considered to be the optimum size for the delivery of personal social services. Social workers feared that they would be dominated by the powerful medical and hospital establishment and the arrangements concerning districts were largely influenced by a desire to reassure them concerning the future of social work services in the new integrated structure.[17] In the event, social work services have held their own very well.

The strictures of the Royal Commission, experience of the working of the structure during the 1970s, and the economic climate of the 1980s have now led to the demise of the district level in favour of the unit of management concept. A study team from Queen's University, reporting in 1976,[18] found that most administrators interviewed thought that the structure did not allow for sufficient delegation, particularly from area to district and that there was confusion in the lines of authority of the district executive team. The 1979 *Consultative Paper* proposed changes at the district or local level with greater delegation of responsibility to strengthen local management delivering hospital and community services. It envisaged units of management based on a reorganisation of the districts. It claimed that the number of districts had led to manning difficulties, imposed considerable burdens on Area Executive Teams and produced undue complexity in the decision-making process. The area and district structure had failed to provide efficient local management for large hospital complexes, especially the Royal Victoria Hospital in Belfast.

In April 1982 the Eastern Health and Social Services Board, with its headquarters in Belfast, rejected the unit of management concept as much too complex to give promise of being effective. In the case of this Board, six districts would give way to some twenty-five units of management. A difference of approach is evident between doctors and administrators with regard to the abolition of districts in favour of units of management. Doctors, wanting strong management at operational level, favoured the introduction of units of management; board members and administrators, anxious about the prospect of diminished spans of control, were in favour of retaining the district structure.

The view has been expressed by District Administrative Officers that there is no substantial evidence to suggest that the structure introduced in 1973 is to blame for these failures but that the failures of the existing structure are related more directly to people's attitudes towards it.[19] There has been a tendency for staff at district level to push queries and problems upwards and to avoid taking responsibility for their resolution. The districts have been denied many of the decisions that would be appropriate to their responsibilities defined under the 1972 guidelines. For example, staff cannot be appointed without the approval of the Area Executive Team, districts cannot undertake minor capital works projects and have no discretion in the use of growth funds. The Area Executive Teams consequently became involved more and more in decisions that ought to have been taken at district level; the tendency to retain responsibility at higher levels confused the roles of district and area staff and removed decisions from service delivery points.

The changes in the structure that were announced in June 1981 are intended to make possible more effective and economical planning and management arrangements by making a clear separation between the roles of chief officers and those involved in unit management. One of the disappointments of the 1973 reorganisation was that chief officers became too involved in operational matters to the detriment of their strategic planning and policy-making functions. The new arrangements emphasise delegation of management decisions to officials at the operational level with no intermediate tier of management between them and Chief Officers at area level. Those responsible for the administration of the unit of management will be professionally and directly responsible to officers at area level and will, in general, have no corporate identity.

The principal changes relate to the role of Chief Officers, to the composition of Area Executive Teams, the replacement of the district level by the unit of management, and the forsaking of the programme of care concept.

Following the 1982 reorganisation Chief Officers are individually accountable to the Board and the corporate responsibilities of AET are limited to those subjects where corporate decisions are essential, for example, advice to the Board on policies, priorities and programmes, and concerning resource allocation. Responsibility for coordination rests with the Chief Administrative Officer and, although he does not have any administrative authority over other chief officers, his role as Secretary to the Board and as Finance Officer places him in a unique position of influence.

Medical representation on the AET is being strengthened by the addition of two further members, a representative of hospital consultants and a representative of general practitioners. The medical advisory machinery which was set up in 1973 has proved to be inadequate mainly because general practitioners, who of course are independent contractors and not employed by boards, felt themselves to be inadequately represented by the chairman of the medical advisory committee. The new arrangements will, it is hoped, help to strengthen links between family doctors and Boards and will assist in planning and delivering community services. It is possible that in the future the presence of three doctors on the AET, where other professions have only one representative, may lead to interprofessional tensions which could make necessary the intervention of the Board. During the summer of 1981 the new arrangements were amended to include the Chief Dental Officer and the Area Pharmaceutical Officer as additional members of the AET and as equal participants with the other members of the Team whenever issues affecting the planning, development, management and control of their services are under consideration.

Despite the modifications which have been seen to be necessary, it must be recorded that many AETs and DETs worked very well indeed from 1973 to 1982 and their success exceeded the early hopes of the architects of the system. Much more, however, could have been achieved if an effective planning service had been introduced much earlier and if more effective political leadership had been available in the first few crucial years and if more high quality administrators had been available to fill the many senior posts created by the reorganisation. Moreover, large numbers of staff were not adequately inducted into the new structure.

Medical advisory machinery

As noted earlier the medical advisory machinery established in Northern Ireland following reorganisation in 1973 was not successful. In addition to major weaknesses at central level, it was ineffective in communicating to Area Executive Teams the views of both family doctors and hospital consultants. Equally, it was often unable to obtain commitment from these groups of doctors to policies framed by AETs. Following the *Report* of the Royal Commission on the National Health Service the Chief Medical Officer was asked to review the workings of the machinery and make recommendations for change.[20]

The main proposal is for a smaller Central Medical Advisory Committee with two standing sub-committees, one for hospital services and one dealing with community medical services. Each of these sub-committees would include the appropriate hospital consultant and community AET representative together with the Chief Administrative Medical Officers of the four Area Boards, representatives of various university and statutory medical agencies. The Hospital Services Advisory Committee would, in turn, be supported by ten proposed speciality committees representative of medical specialties but meeting only once or twice each year.

The committee structure is to be repeated at unit of management level with a Hospital Medical Staff Committee and a Community Medical Committee. A major function of these committees will be to mandate the consultant and community medical members of the Area Executive Team and it is hoped that, through time, this linkage of doctors with the managerial and administrative machinery will make possible more effective planning, coordination and delivery of services.

Public participation: area boards and district committees

The original proposal to establish Health and Social Service Boards implied a reduction in direct public participation and public accountability. The 1969 Green Paper acknowledged that such participation would be substantially reduced under the new proposals. Elected representatives would make up only one-third of the membership of the area boards through nominations by the new district councils. In recommending the removal of major local services, including health and personal social services, from local authority control the Macrory Review Body paid major attention to the responsibilities of the Stormont parliament. Responsibility for health and personal social services would be vested in the appropriate Stormont department and the minister would be accountable to the Stormont Parliament for satisfactory administration. The Macrory Report also envisaged that when these functions became the responsibility of Stormont and the number of councillors was greatly reduced citizens would turn to their Stormont MPs for advice and the redress of grievances. Thus democratic control over the new system would be achieved through overall supervision by the regional parliament. In the middle of the introduction of the legislation to set up the new system the Stormont Parliament was abolished. This has meant that the new system was left without the centrepiece of parliamentary control within Northern Ireland. Responsibility for health and social services rests instead with a junior minister in the Northern Ireland Office and the only element of parliamentary control is through the Westminster Parliament.

The relationship between the boards and the public has been unsatisfactory. Boards are not regarded as representing the community that they serve but as remote and often inaccessible instruments of government policy. The public image of boards reflects a lack of understanding of boards' responsibilities and accountability to the community. Local council representatives are in a minority position and have not been happy with what they see as a lack of decision-making powers in the hands of area boards. On the other hand, criticism has been made of elected representatives concerning their lack of knowledge of the detailed workings of health and personal social services. For example, elected representatives on area boards may be called upon, as employers, to take part in formal procedures dealing with dismissals and personnel matters. Such considerations led to proposals in 1981 that the Minister rather than district councils should nominate which councillors were to serve on area boards from a list of possible members supplied by the District Councils. This proposal received a great deal of criticism from councillors who tended to see it as a way for the Department to get rid of troublesome elected representatives and the idea was subsequently dropped. The 1979 *Consultative Paper* noted that the membership of Health Boards in Britain was smaller than in Northern Ireland and stated its wish to move to smaller boards.[21] In Scotland Boards have from fourteen to twenty-two members and about twenty members are proposed for the new District Authorities in England.

To provide a more direct element of public participation a system of seventeen District Committees similar to the English Community Health Councils was established. District Committees are appointed by the Area Boards and membership includes District Councillors, representatives of voluntary organisations, churches, trade unions and community groups. Area Boards invite nominees from local voluntary groups and other local interests. The District Committees have no executive powers but have the general function of representing and protecting the interests of the public and of commenting on the quality of services. They can offer suggestions for the improvement of services, visit hospitals and homes and report on standards, encourage the activities of voluntary bodies and consider and comment on proposals for development or changes in services. Reports and recommendations of the District Committee are sent to the District Executive Team and the Area Executive Team. District Officers from the District Executive Team attend District Committee meetings, as appropriate, to answer questions and explain policies. The District Committees are dependent on the Area Boards for administrative and secretarial support and have no budget.

There is little sign that District Committees have developed an effective role. Their members have expressed frustration at their impotence and inability to make their voice heard. They have made little impact upon the public and public knowledge of their operations is slight. Their title often leads to them becoming confused with local government administrative districts and their District Councils. The network of voluntary and community groups in Northern Ireland has developed enormously during the last ten years and the District Committee is one of the few ways in which representatives of these groups can link into the statutory framework.

The 1979 *Consultative Paper* showed no awareness of the problems of participation, simply noting that a reduction in the number of districts would require a reduction in the number of District Committees. In the Department's view, there would have been advantages in reorganising the Committees on an area rather than a district basis. Subsequently the Review Group noted that there had been an overwhelming rejection of the suggestion that District Committees might be replaced by Area Committees. The government circular states that committees representative of consumer interests will be retained but their number and composition will be reviewed in the light of the new management structure.

District Committees have formed themselves into an Association of District Committees which may help improve their influence and image to some extent but the District Committee system introduced in 1973 has not really provided for effective participation. Whereas the District Committees in Northern Ireland are also responsible for evaluating the personal social services and representing clients' interests the problems which they have experienced regarding effectiveness and lack of independence are similar to those experienced by the Community Health Councils in Great Britain although Community Health Councils appear to have rather more influence as their representatives can attend Board meetings and participate in planning groups.

Professional integration

Before the 1973 reorganisation took place there was considerable speculation about the relationships that would develop between the professions. Social work, it was feared, would be dominated by medicine;[22] nursing, it was thought, would find it difficult to develop an independent voice and lacked experience in management. Administrators would continue to hold the purse strings and might be reluctant to share their authority.

The Area Executive Team was intended to operate on a corporate or consensus basis. The social work profession, originally apprehensive of medical domination, was given certain guarantees and a statutory personal social services committee to encourage its members to participate. In practice neither the worst fears of social workers or nurses nor what were suspected to be the best hopes of administrators and doctors were realised. Nursing administration is still comparatively underdeveloped (arising from the fact that Northern Ireland introduced the recommendations of the Salmon Committee rather later than elsewhere in the United Kingdom), but there is no evidence that nursing has been a casualty of reorganisation. On the contrary it is probably true to say that reorganisation has provided the nursing profession with new opportunities which it has been slow to exploit.

Social work gained from reorganisation through the creation of more senior posts and better career prospects. Social work directors have had to fight within Area Executive Teams for money, but since 1973 personal social services have enjoyed a high growth rate in terms of available new money. Financially, reorganisation has benefited social work because personal social services departments are no longer dependent on local authority financing as in Great Britain. Many social work facilities had been poorly provided for prior to the 1973 reorganisation by comparison with medical facilities, and, because little money was spent on large new capital projects such as hospitals between 1973 and 1978, money was available for clearly identifiable needs in the personal social services.[23]

No doubt corporate management had some weaknesses in operation, particularly in encouraging delays and the postponement of difficult decisions. Corporate action demanded great changes in attitude from staff who had spent the greater part of their working lives in the traditional model of management. Recent comments on corporate management by the DHSS in Northern Ireland indicate a movement away from the principle. The Review Group quote the Royal Commission on the National Health Service which has pointed to the risk that consensus management could sap individual managerial and professional responsibility. The Review Group stated:

> Both Board and Team members should ensure that the personal responsibilities of individual offices are not blurred or qualified by their responsibilities as members of the Team and that matters which do not require corporate decisions are not unnecessarily referred to the Team. Only in respect of its joint responsibilities – the formulation of advice to the Board on area-wide policies, priorities and programmes together with resource allocation and determining how decisions of the Board should be implemented – should the Team operate by consensus.

The Review Group recommendations for the proposed Unit Management Groups to replace District Executive Teams stated that

> We also recommend that Boards should be given discretion to propose that, where – but only where – circumstances clearly so require, Unit Management Groups should operate in a corporate fashion within guidelines set by the Board.

The *Departmental Circular* endorses this more traditional approach stating that Chief Officers of the Area Boards will be accountable individually to their Boards for the performance of their professional responsibilities and the management of services. The Area Executive Team will be jointly responsible to its Board for certain corporate activities, e.g. policy formulation, planning, resource allocation and monitoring of services. The Circular goes so far as to state that the District Management Group will *not* operate corporately unless the Board so directs.

Northern Ireland social workers have expressed concern that the 1982 administrative reorganisation was inspired by problems in the management of the health service in England. The Northern Ireland pattern, they point out, is different. Northern Ireland has an integrated structure and they fear that the unit of management concept, as it is likely to be applied there, will be hospital, or facility, based and that the community dimension is likely to be diminished by the new arrangements. And they stress that the guidelines on units of management issued to Health and Social Service Boards by the Department of Health and Social Services (Northern Ireland) are virtually identical to those issued by the Secretary of State for Health in England and have a strong emphasis on groupings of hospitals as the basis for the new units. There is little evidence that the special features of the integrated structure in Northern Ireland received adequate emphasis when consideration was being given to the implementation of the unit of management concept in Northern Ireland.

Social workers favour retaining the existing geographical arrangements and their professional orientation tends to stress planning for patient and client groups rather than on the basis of administrative priorities. They also fear that the new management arrangements at AET level, and in particular the strengthening of medical representation there, will dilute the effectiveness of the social work contribution at the most senior level of management and hence right throughout the service.

The new Boards are to be given the freedom to establish such committees as they consider appropriate, making possible the abolition of the statutory Personal Social Services Committee.

The integration of health and personal social services

There is little evidence available to enable an assessment of the impact of the 1973 integration on the standard of services provided.[24] The new structure has certainly provided for closer relationships and better co-ordination between health care and community and social services. Medical personnel may be more aware of the range of community facilities in the area, hostels, day centres, etc., and will more readily understand how community services fit into the overall pattern of care. Social workers may have better access to medical support and para-medical services. It has been argued that the social work challenge to the medical model of care has already had beneficial effects on the care of the mentally handicappped. Improved continuity of care particularly, between hospital and community care, is one of the main tests of integration. This involves integration between hospital and community health services as well as social services. In 1976, for example, the Northern Board reported the efforts of hospital and community nurses to come together to provide an improved integrated nursing service. In some districts this takes the form of joint nursing officer meetings to try to resolve common problems and ensure continuity of care. There have also been attempts to provide a fully integrated maternity service.

In 1973 existing hospital social work departments were amalgamated within the new district social services structure. This should have provided a more effective link with community social services through their involvement in district social services, but it is not clear that it has led to greater use of community facilities. Some demarcation disputes remain. The development of a psychiatric community nursing service has been seen as undermining the role of social workers. The desirability of permanent nursing posts in residential homes and the question of to whom they are responsible has led to controversy between nursing and the personal social services. It is not clear that the medical profession has made a meaningful commitment to working in an integrated way with the other professions.

While integration of services and care may be limited the actual standard of personal social services has improved since reorganisation. The number of qualified social workers has increased substantially. Perhaps the main achievement has been a correction of the uneven balance of services, which had existed prior to the 1973 reorganisation, particularly in the West and in Belfast. Boards have also acted to ensure an equalisation of resources and services throughout their own areas. Planning guidelines issued by the Department encourage a uniform level of provision.

The actual integration of the personal social services with the health services remains more problematic however. This integration was originally intended to be implemented through 'programmes of care'. This concept provided for planning of the management and delivery of services on the basis of identified needs of patient and client groups and was a central component in the whole reorganisation package. Programmes of care never developed as a basis for the organisation and delivery of services. Two of the Boards have established programmes of care teams but they operate on a limited basis. The largest board, the Eastern Board, defines a programme of care as the manpower, facilities, equipment and other resources directed towards providing care to meet the defined needs of an identifiable group in the community. There are four teams of officers appointed on a multi-disciplinary basis and responsible to the Area Executive Team for the preparation of programmes of care in relation to care of the elderly, the care of children and young persons, care of the mentally handicapped and mental health care.

In practice the Eastern Board's programme planning teams have operated as multi-disciplinary groups producing policy advice on multi-disciplinary problems or future needs. The care of the elderly team has examined information on services for old people, nursing care in residential accommodation and day centres. The care of children team has made a survey of the needs of the physically handicapped to assist in the future planning of the service. The mental health programme of care has adopted an integrated approach in advocating a policy of flexible utilisation of services so that a programme of progressive patient care during the various stages of recovery could be established.

The Western Board also has programme planning teams for the elderly, child care, the mentally handicapped, the mentally ill, and the physically handicapped. As well as producing reports on specific future strategies, for example home help services and nursing in residential homes, these teams consider Departmental reports and survey provision.

The programme of care experiment may be said to have failed in Northern Ireland; it is unfortunate that it should have done so, but its lack of success is probably attributable more to lack of political and professional will than to any inherent weakness in the original conception. As an attempt to orientate services to the needs of patient and client groups it was an imaginative initiative. It would be unrealistic to expect it to have been successful at a time of dwindling real resources, undiluted professional autonomy and less than wholehearted commitment to planning on the part of the Area Boards. Members of the programme planning teams had not been adequately equipped to carry out their functions. Assistant chief officers at area level had been recruited to fill a planning function. Failure by chief officers to delegate adequately to district level meant that their assistants were given a service responsibility and this limited their capacity to give the crucial planning function its proper priority within their overall duties. Further, the relationship between districts and the programme planning teams was never clearly defined.

On the positive side there have been some undoubted benefits in terms of the degree of cooperation between the professions in the Executive Team structure, programmes of care, joint study groups on subjects such as child abuse and alcoholism and, occasionally, multi-disciplinary initiatives, for example the establishment of a multi-disciplinary District Adoption Assessment Teams for the physically handicapped in their homes. But there is much less enthusiasm for integration in the chilly economic circumstances of the early 1980s than ten years earlier when the new structure was established.

Conclusion

The 1973 reorganisation has clearly not fulfilled the dreams of its architects of producing a fully integrated system of health and social care. Progress to establishing programmes of care has been limited, but coordination and continuity of care has improved somewhat between hospital and community services. However, teamwork by the disciplines concerned in planning and delivering of services has made only limited progress below Area and District Executive Team level and will be further discouraged by the 1982 restructuring of the management system at district (unit of management) level.

The Royal Commission on the National Health Service accepted the evidence from Northern Ireland that the integration of health and personal social services had been worthwhile and should continue. This evidence (para 16.27) stated that the job of planning health and personal social services had been made simpler and more effective. Total resources could be more easily allocated through the PARR formula.[25] Services could be planned without recourse to the more difficult exercises of joint-funding and joint-planning. Finance and resource allocation decisions for the personal social services are not left with the local authorities where they can be influenced by local political decisions or where the social services have to compete with the needs of large housing or education departments.

Substantive changes in professional relationships and attitudes take a long time to come about. But professional integration has indeed made some progress since the early 1970s, although administrative structures reinforce the fortified positions of the professions and family doctors as independent contractors are, strictly speaking, outside the formal system. The structure has also failed to give the patient and client the centrality they deserve or to provide an effective method of public participation. It has been argued[26] that current preoccupation with bureaucratic structures and the concentration of management techniques have led to neglect of coordination and planning at the primary level. Planning and integration at the point of delivery of service has been consistently neglected and opportunities to improve the quality of service to patients and clients through grass roots integration and coordination have received little encouragement and support. One lesson for the future may be that structural and attitudinal change should be pursued both at the macro and the micro level. The programme of care concept lay at the heart of the decision to bring health and social care services together in 1973; commitment to make it a reality, and to introduce it at different levels throughout the service, could have led to a much greater degree of integration between health and personal social services with all the benefits to patients, clients and staff which that would have brought.

Postscript

In January 1983 the Department of Health and Social Services in Northern Ireland issued Circular HSS(P) 1/83 setting out the unit of management arrangements, their geographical boundaries and senior management structures.

Notes

1. Social Services (Agreement) Act (Northern Ireland), 1949.
2. *The re-shaping of local government: statement of aims*, Belfast: HMSO, 1967, Cmd. 517; *The re-shaping of local government: further proposals*, Belfast: HMSO, 1969, Cmd. 530.
3. *The Administrative Structure of the Health and Personal Social Services in Northern Ireland*, Belfast: HMSO, 1969.
4. For an analysis of the managerial thinking and political and professional influences which culminated in the 1974 reorganisation in England see the excellent paper by Andy Alaszewski, Philip Tether, and Harry McDonnel of the Institute for Health Studies at Hull University: 'Another dose of managerialism? a commentary on the Consultative Paper, *Patient's First*', in *Social Science and Medicine*, Vol. 15A, 1981, pp. 3–15.
5. *Review Body on Local Government in Northern Ireland*, Belfast: HMSO, 1970, Cmd. 546.
6. *Consultative document on the restructuring of the personal health and personal social services in Northern Ireland*, Belfast: HMSO, 1971.

7. Permanent Secretary of the Department of Health and Social Service,, Northern Ireland, 'The restructuring of the social services', Portstewart, 5 May 1971.
8. Booz, Allen and Hamilton, *An integrated service: the re-organisation of health and personal social services in Northern Ireland*, 2 vols., February 1972.
9. Belfast: HMSO, 1975.
10. *The Report of the Royal Commission on the National Health Service* Cmnd. 7615. London: HMSO, 1979.
11. *Consultative Paper on the Structure and Management of the Health and Personal Social Services in Northern Ireland*, Belfast: HMSO, 1979.
12. Chief Medical Officer, *Medical participation and advice in the management of the health and personal social services in Northern Ireland: a review aimed at effectiveness*, Belfast: Department of Health and Social Services, October 1981.
13. Department of Health and Social Services, Departmental Circular HSS (P) 1/81, 'The Structure and Management of Health and Personal Social Services in Northern Ireland', June 1981; see also amending circular, August 1981.
14. *Report of Advisory Group on the Structure and Management of Health and Personal Social Services in Northern Ireland*, Belfast: Department of Health and Personal Social Services, February 1981.
15. 'The Structure and Management of Health and Personal Social Services in Northern Ireland', op cit.
16. For a discussion of the special problems of the North and West District of the Eastern Health and Social Services Board see Arthur Williamson and John Darby, 'Social Welfare Services', in Darby and Williamson (eds.), *Violence and Social Services in Northern Ireland*, London: Heinemann Educational Books, 1978.
17. The British Association of Social Workers, Northern Ireland Region, *The re-organisation of the personal social services*, 1971.
18. J. A. Bates *et al.*, *The reorganization of health and personal social services in Northern Ireland*, Belfast: Department of Business Studies, Queen's University, 1976.
19. Tom Frawley, *The District Administrators' Response to the Consultative Paper on the Structure and Management of the Health and Personal Social Services in Northern Ireland* (Privately published, n.d., 1981); James Lamb, 'Comments on the Consultative Paper on the Structure and Management of Health and Personal Social Services in Northern Ireland' (unpublished, 1981).
20. *Medical participation and advice in the management of the health and personal social services in Northern Ireland*.
21. *Consultative Paper on the Structure and Management of the Health and Personal Social Services in Nortnern Ireland*, op cit.
22. *The reorganisation of the personal social services*.
23. Douglas Smyth, 'The Ulster Scene', unpublished paper, 1977; 'Corporate management in theory and practice', unpublished paper, 1977.
24. Malcolm Brown, 'The dubious advantages of integration', in *Social Work Today*, Vol. 10, no. 27, 6 March 1979.
25. PARR is a resource allocation formula for Northern Ireland similar to RAWP in England.
26. Brian Caul and Stanley Herron, 'A service for people: origins and development of the personal social services of Northern Ireland', printed at the Ulster Polytechnic and privately published by the authors, n.d.

9 Health and Personal Social Services in the United Kingdom: inter-organisational behaviour and service development

John Tibbitt

Introduction

My concern in this paper is with the interaction between health and personal social services agencies over the planning and development of their services. I intend not so much to chart the variety of organisational arrangements which have been created for this purpose although some description of these will be given: rather, I wish to concentrate on the implications of these arrangements for the extent and quality of joint-working which can be expected. The arrangements in Scotland, England and Wales, and Northern Ireland will be discussed in relation to a framework derived from aspects of the sociology of organisations. This discussion leads, in turn, to the identification of topics where a 'within UK' comparative approach might be particularly rewarding both for the study of social policy and for a more complete understanding of the factors influencing inter-organisational transactions more generally.

In common with many other areas of social policy, policies for health and personal social services and for the population groups such as the elderly, the mentally handicapped, and children who constitute the major users of these services, place great stress on collaboration, integration, and the development of a comprehensive range of services. This emphasis can be seen as a response to a variety of factors, some social-demographic, some professional, and some economic. The changing age structure of the population and changes in patterns of morbidity have produced increasing numbers of people requiring longer-term care for chronic conditions rather than intensive treatment for acute illness. This, when seen alongside the wide recognition that the root cause of much of modern illness lies as much with the reaction of the individual to his life situation as it does with organic disease, and that health and social services agencies share a considerable proportion of the same users, has drawn attention to the desirability of a multi-disciplinary approach to the resolution of many presented problems. Professional literature has argued the benefits for service staff from joint working through the opportunities it provides for broad-based preventive care, and for users through improved continuity of care and access to a wider range of services. In economic terms, benefits are expected from more efficient planning and deployment of scarce and often expensive resources.

The reorganisation of health and social work services throughout the United Kingdom in the early 1970s was carried out with an explicit intention, *inter alia*, of facilitating the more efficient planning and development of services. Reorganisation was not directly about patient care but about management and efficient administration, although indirectly this would, it was held, lead to improved quality care. Services were regrouped on the basis of the skill of the service providers: in Scotland and in England and Wales medical and nursing services were grouped into newly constituted health authorities, and social work and related services into new departments of local authorities, whilst in Northern Ireland both groups of services became the responsibility of a single area authority. Reorganisation by skill at a time of increasing emphasis on the multi-disciplinary approach to health and social problems served to bring into sharp focus the need for close collaboration between the services whilst, ironically, making its achievement all the more problematic.

This general concern with the complementary nature of health and social work services has been reflected in a variety of ways in the legislation which effected the reorganisation of services. The National Health Service (Scotland) Act 1972 imposes a duty on local authorities to provide a social work service to the health service and on Health Boards to provide medical assistance to local authorities. Both health and local authorities are required to designate senior officers responsible for liaison between the services, but other mechanisms for joint working such as Joint Liaison Committees (JLCs) and Programme Planning Groups (PPGs), whilst recommended in central government reports, are established at the discretion of the authorities concerned.

In England and Wales, the National Health Service Reorganisation Act 1973, in addition to the duty to mutually assist each other, stipulates a more extensive machinery for collaboration which requires the establishment of Joint Consultative Committees at Area Health Authority level and Health Care Planning Teams (HCPTs), now renamed in some areas Joint Care Planning Teams (JCPTs) at Health District level. The JCCs were given ambitious aims:

> to examine jointly the needs of each area, the plans of the two sets of authorities for meeting needs and the progress made towards meeting them; and to advise on both the planning and operation of the services of common interest.

The objective of the arrangement was

> to secure genuinely collaborative methods of working throughout the planning process, and close and continuing cooperation between officers of both sides.[2]

In Northern Ireland closer links still were introduced through the Health and Personal Social Services (Northern Ireland) Order 1972 which grouped all health and social work services into, in each locality, a single organisation which is corporately managed under the guidance of central government by an Area Executive Team (AET) composed of a Chief Administrative Medical Officer, a Chief Administrative Nursing Officer, a Director of Social Services, and a Chief Administrative Officer. The responsibilities of the AET include the assessment of the needs of the area for coordinated services, developing programme objectives and coordinated plans, allocating resources to districts, and monitoring and evaluating services.

The current programme of restructuring, though taking somewhat different forms in the various parts of the UK is intended to improve further the efficiency of management of the National Health Service. In Northern Ireland the changes are relatively minor involving the extending of corporate management through the augmentation of the AET, and some relocation of responsibility for policy-making. In England and Wales the changes are more significant involving the abolition of the area tier of management and responsibility for the management and delivery of services being placed on newly constituted District Health Authorities. In Scotland some changes are being made in multi-district Health Boards. The duties to collaborate remain as before: however the removal of the conterminosity between area health authority and local social services authority will carry more important implications for the practice of collaboration between them.

The statutory relationship between health and social work services is thus very different in the various constituent parts of the United Kingdom. In Scotland separate health and social work authorities have a duty to collaborate but considerable discretion in the means by which they do so; in England and Wales, in addition to the duty to collaborate, some means for doing so are prescribed; in Northern Ireland, the agencies themselves have been combined. To explore the significance of these differences is one of the major concerns in the discussion which follows. However, before moving on to this, two further points should be made.

First, in keeping with the managerial basis of reorganisation, legislation has been primarily concerned with mechanisms for the strategic planning and development of services in order to avoid duplication and ensure new schemes form part of a well-considered whole. But the efficient integration of services requires collaboration to occur in other spheres as well. In particular, collaboration is necessary over problems of operational management – the sharing of resources to produce the better utilisation of plant and equipment, and in the day-to-day delivery of coordinated patient/client care by practitioners. Factors affecting behaviour over these aspects of the interface between services must also find a place in any discussion of inter-organisational behaviour over the development of services.

The second point relates to the notion of collaboration itself. Despite frequent references to the desirability of collaborative working in both official and professional literature, very rarely is any attempt made to clarify, except in the most general terms, the character of the relationship which is sought. For the purposes of this paper, collaboration is used as an 'umbrella' term referring to a range of possible relationships involving some degree of joint activity by the services concerned, from a minimum requirement of any collaborative relationship that the parties concerned merely share information through to the extreme merger situation in which the parties combine to form a new organisation or service. The various degrees of collaboration can be ordered along a continuum according to the following scheme, based on a typology suggested by Davidson:

> *Communication/consultation* – interaction consists of no more than talking together, sharing information, and informing the other of decisions and developments of mutual interest;
>
> *Cooperation* – a situation in which parties agree to a common, usually high-level or 'banner' goal involving a general undertaking to 'work together', but in which the relationship is marked by a high degree of informality and lack of precision in the operational goals of each service or the means by which activities of the respective parties contribute to the generally desired 'direction';
>
> *Coordination* – arrangements have become more formalised and the tasks of each party more defined. Resources are programmed to take account of each other's separate development plans, but there are no sanctions for non-participation in the collaborative arrangements;
>
> *Integration/teamwork* – a situation in which the parties to a joint-working relationship have more precisely defined tasks and goals, and there are clear arrangements through which it is intended action should take place. The parties act on the basis of common policies and priorities to produce mutually agreed plans. This level of collaboration is characterised by a willingness to concede autonomy to some joint structure and to accept some accountability to it;
>
> *Merger* – in which the separate parties give up their separate identities to form a new organisation.[3]

It is possible to conceive, at least at the theoretical level, of what I will call a 'collaboration profile' relating type and quality of collaboration across the interface between any particular pair of service organisations. The profile can be represented diagrammatically, as shown in Table 9.1.

In the last resort, collaborative activity is 'played out' through the actions of those individuals concerned with each type of collaboration.

Table 9.1 Hypothetical collaboration profile between service organisations

Type of collaboration	*Quality of collaboration*				
	Com.	Coop.	Coord.	Int.	Merger
Strategic planning/development					
Operational management					
Service delivery to clients					

Each person who undertakes these activities does so as an occupant of a number of statuses: as a member of an administrative organisation, as a member of a profession, as an individual with his own particular set of attitudes and expectations, and as a member of small work groups composed of those from other organisations also involved in particular collaborative activities. These are not listed in any particular order – indeed it is to be expected that, as each type of collaborative activity takes place in different settings and under different conditions, the relative importance of the various statuses will be related to the type of activity being undertaken. I will now introduce a framework that will identify variables which are liable to influence behaviour in each of these statuses, and which when related to particular situations may suggest or account for variations in the 'shape' of collaboration profiles.

Theoretical perspectives

Let us start from a position which would regard the interface between health and social work services as being concerned essentially with the inter-organisational relationships between two sets of large complex organisations, namely area (or district) health authorities and local authority social work and social services departments.

The orthodox approach to the study of organisations regards them as 'social units (or human groups) deliberately constructed and reconstructed to seek specific goals'.[4] The specific goals and the functions that they lead the organisations to undertake for their realisation constitute what Levine and White have called the 'organisational domain'.[5] It is the principal concern of the management of an organisation to protect or expand its domain by taking steps to ensure the continuing performance of functions at the present level or to increase the level of performance or gain new functions. The ability to extend the organisational domain will depend upon the acquisition of further resources which may range from material goods and skilled personnel to social prestige. Such resources are usually scarce, placing organisations in competition with others and dependent on the actions of others within their environment. The ways in which an organisation manages its dependence on its environment is therefore crucial for an understanding of organisational behaviour.

Dill has labelled the primary elements of an organisation's environment as its 'organisation set', which is composed of the focal organisation's funders and suppliers, regulatory bodies, clientele, and other agencies with related goals.[6] The means by which an organisation may attempt to manage its dependency on others in its organisation set has received only a limited amount of attention in the literature. Thompson and McEwan argue that organisations may adopt one or a combination of several behavioural strategies including 'coalition' (joining with other organisations), 'exchange' (bargaining for resources with other organisations), 'penetration' (the placement of some of its members in other organisations), and 'co-optation' (the incorporation of members of other organisations into its own decision-making structure). The adoption of any particular strategy will depend on a number of variables concerned with the organisation itself (for example, its present resource position, its own method of organisation), and with its environment (for example, the stability of the inter-organisational network, the relative prestige of the organisations involved).[7] Levine and White focus on the exchange process between organisations. They suggest a number of factors which affect the degree of interdependence and hence the likelihood of co-operation and exchange between organisations, namely the extent to which each organisation has access to suitable resources, the relative objectives of the organisations and the functions to which resources are allocated, and the degree to which domain consensus exists between organisations. In a further discussion of inter-organisational cooperation and exchange, Reid has hypothesised a similar set of conditions necessary for significant interaction to occur. These are, first, that the organisations should have shared goals; second, they should have complementary resources; and third, that there should be efficient mechanisms for controlling the exchange process. Reid adds a further hypothesis that the more valuable the resource the more cautious an agency will be in engaging in cooperative ventures.[8]

With respect to the particular interface of interest in this paper, the strategies used to manage interdependency are likely to be greatly influenced by the fact that a crucial element in the resources of each organisation is the professional staff who constitute the majority of its employees. Indeed the management of both organisations is frequently in the hands of those who are both administrators and professionals. The respective characteristics of the dominant professions in health and social work are markedly different. The medical profession has a long history, enjoys high social prestige, and has developed a large body of specialist knowledge. In addition it has a code of ethics and professional practice which is regulated by the profession itself and by which it attempts to control the standards of its members. These factors have placed it in a favourable position to attract further resources, to extend its knowledge and its domain by bringing more and more conditions within the ambit of medical treatment. Social work, on the other hand, is not so favourably placed. It is a new profession still aspiring for professional recognition (some argue social work can never be other than a 'semi-profession').[9] It does not enjoy high social prestige, it has no widely accepted knowledge base, and as yet, no generally accepted codes of ethics or professional practice. Most members are accountable to their employing authorities for the standard of their work, rather than to any central controlling professional body. Successive reorganisations and the extension of legal responsibilities without a commensurate expansion in resources have done nothing for the self-confidence of the profession. These fundamental differences between the professions in material resources, in recognised specialist skills, and in social presitge, have profound implications for any exchange process which may occur between them. These same differences will in turn mediate any interaction between their employing administrative organisations which orthodox organisation theory might otherwise suggest.

But orthodox organisation theory itself has been severely criticised. Difficulties spring from the fundamental concept of a specific organisation goal against which performance can be assessed. Research into the functioning of various organisations has shown that alongside formally declared goals there often exist informal goals; usually organisations have multiple goals which are not always mutually consistent; goals are often diffuse, expressed in general and vague terms; goals even formally expressed may be perceived differently by different members of the organisation; and the goals of an organisation are subject to change. These criticisms have urged an alternative approach. Perrow has pointed out that, strictly speaking, it is the individuals in organisations who have goals and not the organisations themselves,[10] and Bittner has argued that the study of such concepts as 'goal' needs to be based on the investigation of how participants use them as common-sense concepts in the course of their day-to-day behaviour.[11] Thus, whilst orthodox organisation theory serves to draw attention to important dimensions of the interface situation, it is also necessary to focus on the individual worker and to seek to discover the features of the reality in which he operates.

It has already been observed that most members of health and social work services organisations are members also of a profession. The notion of 'professional ideology', by which is meant a set of relatively abstract ideas and attitudes about some ideal performance of a professional role, has been found to be particularly helpful in the study of a variety of welfare agencies. The place of professional ideology in the process of 'constructing reality' has been explored in some detail by Smith who develops a model linking professional ideology with operational philosophies, the administrative system in action, and the subsequent situated accounts of events which actors provide, which themselves will ultimately feed back into professional ideology.[12] For the present purposes, the value of the model lies in alerting research to the need to study the perceptions of their own professional role and that of others held by each actor in the collaborative situation, the ways in which these are operationalised, the ways in which mechanisms for collaboration attempt to cope with the various and sometimes competing operationalisations, and the outcomes which result.

Mention of the mechanisms by which collaboration is attempted draws attention to a further perspective with important implications for the understanding of interaction between agencies. More and more, social services (broadly defined) are planned, delivered, evaluated, and coordinated by multi-professional groups or 'teams'. The multi-professional work-group is, in most cases a face-to-face group which might be expected to function in a similar manner to any other primary group. It is perhaps ironic that although many of the professions involved in the provision of health and social work services would claim some familiarity with group dynamics, the collaboration work group is seldom discussed in these terms. The literature on groups, drawn from a variety of disciplines, focuses on a number of variables which have been shown to be related to group performance such as size, leadership selection and style, decision-making procedures, means of communication, and stability of group membership. A group will seek to impose some norms of behaviour on its members. Group norms will not necessarily be consistent with other norms, for example, professional practice, which members are also likely to hold. An excessive attachment either to group norms or to professional norms may have implications for the individual concerned by rendering him inflexible in his professional work outside the group or by restricting his distinctive professional input to the group that justifies multi-disciplinary working in the first place. The perceived relative positions of members of the group in status and power (which would seem to be clearly felt despite attempts in the health and social services to create 'teams of equals') are likely to be related to adherence to group norms, and will influence the extent and type of contribution to the work of the group made by its various members.

Each of the perspectives outlined above focuses on particular aspects of the social situations in which collaborative activities occur, and together, they serve to illustrate the complexity of the social processes of interaction across organisational boundaries. Using the insights derived from these different approaches, I now want to move on to a discussion of the situations in which the joint development of health and social work services occurs in the different parts of the United Kingdom.

Strategies for the management of dependency

We have already noted that organisations may follow one or a number of strategies in their attempts to maintain an appropriate relationship with other organisations within their environment. Whilst research into the workings of many aspects of the machinery for joint planning and development of health and social services is still sparce, I will draw on some of the available material in order to illustrate the potential utility of the concepts that have been introduced in the foregoing section, and to suggest some areas for further research where a comparative approach might be particularly useful.

Let us pursue, first, the persepctive on inter-organisational behaviour provided by exchange theory. The reorganisation of health and social services can be seen as an attempt to provide more appropriate conditions for exchange between these services. Levine and White have distinguished three main categories of elements which may be exchanged by health and welfare organisations. These are firstly, referrals of cases, clients, or patients; second, the giving or receiving of labour services including professional skills; and third, the sending or receiving of resources other than labour services, particularly funds and information.[13] Here I shall be less concerned with the first of these, and will concentrate on exchange of financial and professional resources.

A device for the provision of financial resources specifically earmarked for the development of services on the boundaries of health and social work is available in England and Wales. First announced in 1976, joint financing is an arrangement allowing the limited use of health services resources in support of local authority spending on projects which can be expected to make a better contribution in terms of total care than if applied to health services directly. The rules allow the health authority to make a substantial contribution (up to 100%) to the capital and revenue costs of projects, the revenue contribution being available on a reducing scale for up to seven years.

The introduction of this scheme had several purposes. The strategy was first aired in 1975 when it was put forward as a suggestion to the Leyfield Committee as a means of fostering collaboration across service boundaries and between the very differently financed health authorities and local authority social services departments by offering a financial incentive to local authorities to collaborate with health authorities. Additionally, the scheme was seen as a means of giving effect to overall government policy of shifting the balance between hospital services and community care, and as a means, at a time of financial constraint, of encouraging the development of services at points where the respective responsibilities of each service overlapped, for example, over the care of frail elderly, the mentally handicapped and the mentally ill.

Despite some initial administrative problems and continuing frustrations arising from the cumbersome nature of joint planning in multi-district health authorities and from the lack of terminosity in some planning areas, in 1979 it was reported that 94% of local authorities took up joint-financing allocations.[14] Joint finance money has been applied to a wide range of projects including mother and child centres, night sitting services, travelling wardens, and laundry services. It is estimated that 27–33% of joint finance expenditure was allocated to projects for the elderly, 31–35% for the mentally handicapped, 7–13% for the mentally ill, 4–5% on the non-elderly physically handicapped and 22–26% on other groups including children. Of schemes costing over £50,000, more than one-quarter were for day centres, and more than half for residential care.[15]

A recent survey by the National Association of Health Authorities in England and Wales has shown wide support amongst health authorities for the continuation of joint funding but reports many experiencing some problems in take-up by their local authorities because of the financial restraints on local government expenditure.[16]

A thorough evaluation of the effect of joint financing is yet to be made, but such assessments as there are would seem to suggest that each of the aims with which the DHSS initiated the scheme has been met to some degree. Thus under this scheme a considerable boost has been given to the services available for a number of client groups who might otherwise have found themselves low in the order of priorities of the individual health and social services authorities acting on their own, and to services located in the community. It is suggested too that the necessity of identifying projects suitable for joint financing has greatly improved relationships between officers of the respective service organisations.

However, whether or not the availability of joint finance has fostered joint planning seems to be open to doubt.[17] As well as its use on 'imaginative' or 'noteworthy' schemes, it has also been used to restore cut services, to bring old capital schemes out of mothballs, and to extend existing basic services. As joint financing offers for many local authorities virtually the only source of growth money, it has been argued that it has been seen as a short-term expedient which has distorted the achievement of longer-term policies for service development. In any case, there seems to be doubt on the extent to which expenditure has been the result of mutually agreed policies and priorities by officers and members of the respective authorities rather than as the outcome of a search based on administrative criteria for existing projects which would seem to fall within the rules of the joint-funding scheme. It does seem though that joint financing has formed the focus of most joint planning activity in England and Wales. Joint planning will take time to develop, and the provision of joint financing has provided local authorities and area health authorities with an important stimulus to learn how to talk to each other constructively in an attitude of cooperation rather than competition. However it remains to be seen whether the fact that the two organisations are organised on such different principles of administration and practice will prevent further progress along the continuum of collaboration leading to close working relationships and the development of plans on the basis of common assumptions. Booth is not optimistic.[18]

In Northern Ireland there ought not to be any need for joint financing as a specific scheme as the planning for all services is carried out on the basis of one common pool of resources. As with joint finance, no systematic monitoring or evaluation of this situation is yet available, although a number of impressionistic assessments have been published. A number of factors are seen as hampering the development of corporate planning. Important among these are the close control exerted by the DHSS(NI) which leaves little scope for action on the part of the area boards, the lack of material available to the boards from programme planning groups, and the functionally-based committee structure through which the boards operate. These latter factors have tended to reinforce service boundaries rather than reduce their significance. Whatever the reasons, Birrell and Williamson (see Chapter 8 of this volume) have concluded that the original intention to plan on a programme basis across services 'has not been brought to birth'.

In Scotland the situation is different again. Whilst it has always been possible for health boards and local authorities jointly to contribute to the funding of projects of mutual benefit to each authority, until recently there was no scheme comparable to the joint funding arrangements in England and Wales to provide additional stimulus to the development of joint planning. Such joint planning and pooling of resources which has occurred has depended on the recognition of other grounds for interaction. Since 1980, a limited scheme of 'support financing' has been introduced whereby a small sum of health service funds is earmarked for use in projects that would normally be regarded as social work projects on a basis similar to the joint funding scheme in England and Wales. It is too early yet to assess the effect of the availability of this support finance on joint planning among Scottish authorities.

These various situations for the availability of finance as one aid to joint planning would appear to present an opportunity of exploring some of the assumptions upon which the theory of inter-organisational exchange is based. Finance is a key resource for the development of any service. Reid emphasised the need for complementary resources as a condition for the development of exchange.[19] The various parts of the UK offer a variety of models: one where until very recently, there has been no common pool of resources, one in which there is a modest supply of transferable resources, and another in which resources are allocated in their entirety from a single pool. Through careful comparative studies of the planning and decision-making processes in each situation, research might seek to discover the effect of the availability of joint finance on joint planning, whether or not it is a necessary condition, and its importance in relation to other factors either structural or concerned with the interaction over the use of other key resources such as professional skill.

I will now move on to the exchange of non-financial resources. The principal means by which professional and management knowledge and skills might be exchanged over the planning process is through the various formal committees which have been established for the purpose in the different parts of the United Kingdom. Once again, research on the functioning of these bodies is still very underdeveloped with the result that it is possible to form only a very tentative view of their operation.

Brown has described the early days in the operation of the Joint Consultative Committee in Humberside.[20] Originally this committee consisted of eight local authority members, mostly from departments of social services, education, and planning, and six area health board members. In addition to the JCC itself, four high level officer groups were established concerned with collaboration, social services, child health, and environmental health and housing, in support. Brown sees a number of achievements of this system, especially for officers. The early benefits included allowing those involved to form a better idea of each other's functions, the discovery that the local authority planning department held a mass of demographic data relevant for health service planning, and steps were taken to see how health authority capital schemes might be better related to strategic plans for community development. However, at member level the JCC does not seem to have been so effective. Lists of capital schemes in health, education and social services were tabled but received little discussion, and very little systematic consideration was given to a number of important issues raised by the collaboration group such as resource saving on transport, catering, and domestic services, or about the provision of social work services to hospitals.

Joint Consultative Committees exist only in England and Wales. Scotland and Northern Ireland have placed reliance on the Programme Planning Group or Committee as a means of fostering collaboration between services. In Scotland the Programme Planning Committees of one of the Area Health Boards have been appraised by Boddy.[21] He found that many of the members, particularly those from nursing, paramedical and local authority services, attached great value to the fact that they were now able to express their professional views on policy matters. For some this value lay in the development of inter-professional relationships itself, although for others it was seen as increasingly unacceptable that their members should be asked to operate policies in the discussion of which they had not been involved. As far as the output of the groups was concerned, Boddy observes that reports tend to list ideally desirable services rather than come to decisions about priorities or preferred alternative strategies which would have involved the groups working through differences in professional viewpoints. The groups' either inability or avoidance of the problems of resolving inter-professional differences was seen as stemming, at least in part, from the fact that the majority of participants in the groups saw themselves primarily in the capacity of representatives of the interests of their own profession or authority.

In many ways similar to the programme planning group is the Health Care Planning Team – a multi-professional group of staff concerned with services to a particular client group, seen as a key component to planning at health district level in England and Wales. Towell comments that the initial enthusiasm for the HCPT has given way to considerable doubts about both the functions and usefulness of such groups.[22] It is not clear whether they in fact function as planning groups or as consultative bodies, whether they should focus on specific district problems or range more widely over the needs of client groups, or whether they should be only pressure groups for low priority services. It appears that many such teams have become less concerned with planning as opposed to more immediate issues of operational coordination. Booth in a recent study of joint care planning in one English area comments that:

> each authority has tended to view the process primarily as a means of helping to resolve some of the pressures on and deficiencies in its own services. . . . The pursuit of narrow organisational interests rather than wider community interests has led to each authority adopting an institutionally defined view of health and social problems which owes more to the administrative division of functions and responsibilities between them than to the nature of community needs.[23]

Despite further central government guidance which has stressed the importance of joint care planning, there remains considerable debate on the functioning of these groups.

From this cursory review of what is in itself a very underdeveloped field of research, there would not appear to be any clear evidence that the mechanisms which have been created to further the development of joint planning and operation of services, ideally to the stage of integration of policies and services, have been particularly effective. We have seen that even where planning has been based on the availability of transferable financial resources or from a common pool there is little evidence that such funds have been disbursed on schemes according to mutually agreed priorities; where joint planning has had to rest on other motivations, whilst information and individual service plans have been exchanged, it would seem that exchange has failed to reach a level where collaboration could be said to have progressed beyond the basic stages of the continuum advanced earlier. In particular, the difficulties of PPGs and HCPTs in formulating common policies, other than statements of ideal situations in which each service gets a share, would seem to indicate the failure of the participating organisation representatives to establish sufficient domain consensus to allow exchange to develop. In coming to a better understanding of each other's roles members may also discover how wide are their differences in approach to the needs of particular population groups.

In this situation it may be that exchange is not the strategy which organisations consider will best meet their own needs, and may therefore choose to pursue others. Brown notes that despite the ineffectiveness of the JCC, considerable collaborative activity occurs outside this formal machinery, through, for example, a 'care of the elderly liaison group', review teams on non-accidental injury to children, and on other groups.[24] It would seem therefore that there is considerable penetration of the health service management machinery by social services staff in an attempt to influence the decision-making of the health service. Again, it should be noted that PPGs and HCPTs are essentially health service bodies which advise health authorities on policy matters. In including social services representatives on them, the health service is arguably following a strategy of co-optation as one means of reducing the possibilities of antithetical actions on the part of the two organisations.

Elkin has suggested that organisations with limited resources in relation to others in their environment are likely to seek to manage dependency through penetration or coalition,[25] whilst Selznick has explored the notion of co-optation.[26] He distinguishes 'formal' co-optation which entails the absorption of elements of other organisations into the host organisation in order to secure their public accountability for decisions but allows them little influence over the actual decision-making process, and 'informal' co-optation which is the converse, sharing in decision-making without accountability for the decisions made. Thus formal co-optation is a strategy for lending legitimacy to decisions reached whilst informal co-optation involves yielding to a source of power. Clearly, whilst analytically distinct, the two forms of co-optation are not mutually exclusive: groups brought in to share responsibility may exploit the access they have gained and encroach on the decision-making process itself.

Further support for the suggestion that a strategy of exchange may not be the most likely one for health or social services to adopt comes from consideration of the relative positions of the professional organisations whose members constitute the essential resources of the respective administrative organisations. In particular the dominance of the medical profession over the control and priorities of the health services now faces challenges from a number of fronts. Changes in the patterns of morbidity render the prevailing mode of medical practice based on high technology based in acute hospitals of diminishing utility, and its associated allocation of priorities increasingly inappropriate. A change of allocation of priorities from the curative approach to one of care involves both a loss in resources to those who have been able previously to determine priorities and greater involvement of other health workers. The conceding of power in the control of treatment situations is not something for which many doctors have been trained nor something which their profession, as an organisation, will easily accept. Whilst medical prestige and priorities continue to be allocated to the ever greater sophistication of acute treatment, resources concerned with prevention, health education, and community health care will not be of much value in the exchange process. Health services may therefore be expected to seek strategies which will contain pressures from others within their environment and attract legitimacy to their decisions.

The different mechanisms through which joint planning and decision-making take place between health and local authorities in the constituent parts of the UK would seem to provide an attractive field in which to study factors leading organisations to the choice of particular strategies in managing their relationships with other organisations within their environment. The formal system of JCCs and HCPTs in England and Wales can be seen as an attempt to create a relationship of 'enforced exchange', but the existing sketchy evidence on the performance of the system throws doubt on the extent to which this strategy has been achieved. In Northern Ireland it remains to be examined whether 'banging heads together'[27] in the management of a unified service leads to mutual involvement or a perpetual struggle of wills for dominance and resources or a corporate collusion to proceed in separate ways. In Scotland the PPG system needs examination, and the reasons for the creation of Joint

Liaison Committees where these have been seen as desirable warrant investigation. They offer health boards, for example, one way of securing the political commitment of local authority members to joint planning deliberations.

The process of interaction

I have been concerned so far with inter-organisational behaviour at the level of the organisation itself, and have attempted to demonstrate ways in which comparative research might use theory at this level as a framework for increasing our understanding of the functioning of health and social services agencies over joint planning. But as I also pointed out earlier, inter-organisational relationships occur through the interactions of individuals, and not only over joint planning but also over the management and delivery of services to individual patients and clients. In order to avoid an over-simplistic view of organisational behaviour it is necessary to devote some attention to the actual processes of interaction which occur as these relationships are 'played out'.

The best developed area of research on the health–social services interface is concerned with transactions between various service professionals in the delivery of services to individual cases. One of the basic interests of this research has been in patterns of communication. Although there is evidence that a considerable amount of communication does take place, studies show that it is frequently perceived as inadequate by those involved, either because of its frequency, direction or content. Obviously successful communication depends on the ready availability of means by which to communicate, but in addition, it will only occur if there is a sufficient degree of consensus among the parties to the communications over the role, functions, and competence of other services.

Research has been largely concerned with these issues. It is clear there is considerable ignorance about the jobs of other services. It is also clear that ignorance has frequently led to prejudice and stereotyping. The literature is replete with quotes from doctors about social workers 'fresh from the barricades of the LSE', wearing 'pink shirts' and 'burst tennis shoes', and similar statements by other professionals. In this situation of limited understanding of others' roles, it has been demonstrated that one service may redefine problems referred to it by other professions[28] and how selection of clientele by other agencies can lead to inappropriate members of the target population receiving services.[29]

The importance of individually held professional ideologies and operational philosophies for inter-professional relationships has also been identified. For example, a study of social workers acting as mental health officers shows clearly the wide variation within this one professional group about the role and tasks deemed appropriate in undertaking this work.[30]

Study of the interaction between social workers and members of primary health care teams shows how particular workers were regarded quite differently by the various members of the team with obvious implications for the collaboration which occurred. Again, research shows clearly that the frequency of interaction between a social worker and the various members of a group of general practitioners differs markedly, and is related to the perceptions held by the GP of what constitutes a social problem suitable for referral and what is his own role in dealing with non-medical aspects of the problems presented to him.

In treating individual cases doctors adhere strongly to an independent professional stance, intended to minimise organisational influences over the actions they choose to take. Social workers, although much more subject to the bureaucratic control of their employing agencies still have considerable freedom over their actions at least in so far as consultation and involvement of others in the case is concerned. At this level it is arguable that the delivery of services depends heavily on the individual orientations of the practitioners involved, organisational policies increasingly intruding as access to resources outside the control of the individual practitioners is required.

The operational management of resources is probably the aspect of inter-organisational behaviour where the inclinations of practitioners and organisations, both professional and administrative, are most sharply juxtaposed. As yet there are very few studies of working groups such as case conferences, multi-disciplinary assessment committees, and district level management or liaison groups. In such groups, members are both representatives of the 'home' organisations with interests which will not be the same as those of other group members, and members of a task-orientated group. This situation creates dilemmas for participants, and the functioning of the group will depend in large measure on how these are handled. The individual member's primary orientation will determine the type of behaviour in which he engages in the group. However, behaviour will also be subject to group pressures, how the group is convened, its leadership, and methods of working will all contribute to its overall performance.

The differences in organisational structure which were the focus of the discussion of joint planning at the strategic level would not be expected to be of such significance at either the case or operational management levels. Similar groups of people will interact over these matters in each of the constituent geographical areas of the UK. However, carefully conceived comparative studies carried out in diverse organisational settings are urgently needed if a more complete understanding of interaction over these aspects of the interface is to be obtained.

In conclusion

A recap of the argument presented here is now appropriate. The early sections of the paper were concerned to demonstrate the interdependence of health and social work services and to describe the legislative response to this through the reorganisations of the services in each part of the UK in the early 1970s. It was pointed out that reorganisation was essentially concerned with the efficient management and planning of the services, mainly at the strategic level, but that effective joint development of services also required collaboration over operational management of resources and between individual practitioners in the delivery of services. It was further emphasised that the notion of collaboration is itself problematic, and can include a wide range of relationships. Given that the various levels of collaboration involve different people and take place in different settings there was a need to look at the quality of collaboration at each level of interaction if a 'profile' of the interface between any particular pair of organisations is to be obtained.

The paper then moves to a discussion of theoretical perspectives which can provide a framework for the analysis of inter-organisational interaction. Three such perspectives were outlined: aspects of the sociology of organisations, elements of an interactionist perspective, and others from the sociology of small groups. Together these draw attention to a number of variables that might be investigated in relation to the situations in which the joint development of health and social work services occurs in the different parts of the UK. In particular, it is concluded that comparative research of the constituent parts of the UK would be appropriate first for an examination of inter-organisational behaviour as exchange and the factors that might be conducive to exchange, and second for the investigation of processes of strategic choice by organisations in managing their dependency on other organisations. The final part of the paper argued that in situations other than high level joint planning the scope for influence of other variables on patterns of inter-organisational relationships which organisation theory would otherwise expect are greatest, and draws attention to the need for comparative research, not necessarily across national boundaries, but between organisational settings to examine the inter-meshing of all these variables on the outcome of interaction across organisational boundaries.

It is one thing to argue the benefits from comparative research on such a basis as this, but quite another to provide a sufficiently precise operationalisation of the rather ill-defined concepts which have been included in this discussion. Nevertheless the framework presented may be found useful as the basis for further work which can operationalise the concepts and test relationships among them. If this can be done, the payoff would be both in a greater understanding of inter-organisational relationships in general, and in the identification of steps which might be taken to further the aims of policies in health and social services in particular.

Notes

1. The opinions expressed in this paper are those of the author. These should not be taken as necessarily representing those of the Scottish Office.
2. *Report from the Working Party on Collaboration Between the NHS and Local Government*, London: HMSO, 1973.
3. S. M. Davidson, 'Planning and Coordination of Social Services in Multi-organisational Contexts', *Social Services Review*, Vol. 50, no. 1.
4. A. Etzioni, *Modern Organisations*, Englewood Cliffs, New Jersey: Prentice Hall, 1964.
5. S. Levine and P. E. White, 'Exchange as a Conceptual Framework for the Study of Inter-organisational Relationships', *Administrative Science Quarterly*, Vol. 5, 1961.
6. W. Dill, 'Environment as an Influence of Managerial Autonomy', *Administrative Science Quarterly*, Vol. 2, 1958.
7. J. D. Thomson and W. J. McEwan, 'Organisational Goals and Environment: Goal Setting as an Interaction Process', *American Sociological Review*, Vol. 28, no. 1, 1958.
8. W. Reid, 'Inter-agency Coordination in Delinquency Prevention and Control', in M. N. Zald (ed.), *Social Welfare Institutions*, New York: Wiley, 1965.
9. A. Etzioni, *The Semi-Professions and the Organisation: Teachers, Nurses and Social Workers*, New York: Free Press, 1969.
10. C. Perrow, *Organisation Analysis: A Sociological View*, London: Tavistock, 1970.
11. E. Bittner, 'The Concept of Organisation', *Social Research*, Vol. 32, no. 3, 1965.
12. G. Smith, 'The Place of Professional Ideology in the Analysis of Social Policy: some theoretical conclusions from a pilot study of the children's panels', *Sociological Review*, Vol. 25, no. 4, 1977.
13. 'Exchange as a Conceptual Framework for the Study of Inter-organisational Relationships'.
14. *Health and Social Services Journal*, 6 April 1979.
15. A. Norton, 'Joint Care and Joint Planning', *Local Government Studies*, Vol. 5, no. 2, 1979.
16. W. Wistow and S. Herd, 'Pump-priming Programme', *Health and Social Services Journal*, 3 July 1981.
17. T. A. Booth, 'The Swings and Roundabouts of Sharing Out Resources', *Health and Social Services Journal*, 25 November 1977.
18. T. A. Booth, 'Collaboration between the Health and Social Services: Part 2, A case study of joint finance', *Policy and Politics*, Vol. 9, no. 2, 1981.
19. 'Inter-agency Coordination in Delinquency Prevention and Control'.
20. R. G. S. Brown, 'Collaboration Between the NHS and Local Government', *Local Government Studies*, Vol. 2, no. 2.
21. D. Boddy, 'Programme Planning Committees of the Greater Glasgow Health Board', *Health Bulletin*, Vol. 35, no. 5.
22. D. Towell, 'Making Reorganisation Work: Challenges and Dilemmas in the Development of Community Medicine', in K. Barnard and K. Lees (eds), *Conflicts in the National Health Service*, London: Croom Helm, 1977.

23. T. A. Booth, 'Collaboration Between the Health and Social Services: Part 1, A case study of joint care planning', *Policy and Politics*, Vol. 9, no. 1, 1981.
24. 'Collaboration Between the NHS and Local Government'.
25. S. L. Elkin, 'Comparative Urban Politics and Inter-organisational Behaviour', *Policy and Politics*, Vol. 2, no. 4, 1974.
26. P. Selznick, *TVA and the Grass Roots*, Berkeley: University of California Press, 1949.
27. As M. Brown in 'The dubious advantages of integration', *Social Work Today*, Vol. 27, no. 10, 1979, puts it.
28. A. Ullman and G. C. Kassebaum, 'Referrals and Services in a Medical Social Work Department', *Social Services Review*, Vol. 35, no. 3, 1961.
29. B. C. Berkman and R. Rehr, 'Early Social Services Case Finding for Hospitalised Patients: an Experiment', *Social Services Review*, Vol. 47, no. 2, 1973.
30. J. E. Tibbitt, *Social Workers as Mental Health Officers*, Edinburgh: HMSO, 1978.

PART THREE
Comparison in Other Fields of Social Policy

10 National and Regional Aspects of Housing Policy and Provision in the United Kingdom

Alan Murie

Introduction

Analysis of housing problems in Britain has moved away from approaches where household characteristics are regarded as central in explaining patterns of stress and inequality. Greater emphasis is now paid to the relationship between housing and other parts of the economy. It is argued that housing problems are not the result of processes that are necessarily specific to the housing market, that housing policy is only one strand of government action which may ameliorate or exacerbate current housing problems and that it is important to examine housing in the context of major features of the process of economic development.

In Britain a major feature of economic restructuring over the last fifty years has been regional differences and persistent spatial differences at that level. Thus it could be concluded that the British housing literature needs to take explicit account of the relationship between housing policies and regional development. Differences in administrative, financial or legislative arrangements should be seen in the context of regional development and inequality. Housing progress and problems are linked with levels of income, unemployment and occupational structure. It is no coincidence that the worst housing conditions in the British Isles occur in Northern Ireland and that other areas with regional economic 'problems' also fall into adverse categories. The implication is that this is not a result of individual or household characteristics or the quality of management and planning but is a product of the pattern of economic development and is indicated by the concentration of low-paid employment, unemployment and low household and per capita income. Crucial questions involve the role of policy (whether it has been the same as in other parts of the UK or different) and analysis of its influence in areas with different problems. These kind of perspectives make the national–regional dimension relevant in its own right. Comparison at a regional–national level ceases to be merely a vehicle for testing hypotheses about the importance of various differences in policy and practice and becomes a central dimension in the relationship between housing and economic development. Housing location in the first instance is determined by industrial and commercial location, and shifts in industrial and commercial activity have clear implications for the relative attraction and value of infrastructure (including houses) in areas made peripheral to economic activity. The social and market processes which operate in different areas are general, and underlie the operation and structure of institutions and decisions about the location and types of dwellings constructed, changes in housing and the nature of state intervention. These general processes are essentially market ones linked with economic change, and are derived from the relationship between housing and other aspects of economic change. Consequently, a crucial element in understanding housing issues and housing policy in Britain is explanation and analysis that relate housing to uneven economic development, and national–regional economic circumstances to housing policy and practice.

The development of research in Britain has not been marked by any sustained or substantial regional or conurbation focus. One reason for this, it could be argued, is that research which is to be relevant for policy must have a local authority rather than a regional focus. If we assume that the need for research has been accepted, and that the limitations of national aggregate material are evident, what types of research are most relevant? The present emphasis in official study is with local authorities, reflecting the preoccupation with policy analysis. Local authorities are the implementers of policy, and it is their practice and exercise of discretion which determines the effect of much of housing policy. However, it is clear that markets and processes do not pay attention to administrative boundaries. Regional differences in house prices, house conditions, the age and tenure structure of the housing stock, employment and economic circumstances and associated levels of housing demand, migration, housing shortage and housing stress mean that policy measures have different effects in different areas and that 'problems' of the household or the administration differ in different areas.

Housing is a fixed capital investment with a high cost and long life and the nature of the housing market and dominance of market relationships affects the nature of public intervention. The public sector does not have any monopoly of provision and does not control the standard or nature of service provision. Indeed it is heavily constrained by market forces in matters of cost and price. This is a different set of circumstances than apply in other social policy areas and may result in the spatial dimension being considerably more important. It is not necessary to argue further that there is a local and regional dimension to policy. The differences that exist at this level are important and both explanations of difference and proposals for intervention require evidence at a regional and local level if they are to have any substance. However, what is appropriate for this paper is to consider the wider relevance of comparative study. The experience of housing policy and housing research suggests that local and regional evidence is necessary if policies in those localities and regions are to be relevant. But there are other considerations that indicate the value of comparisons for broader purposes.

The national–regional dimension and comparative study

There is a considerable and growing literature concerned with comparison of housing situations, housing administration or housing policy in different countries. Much of this literature falls into the category of historical description and statements about key legislation. There is an absence of any clear framework for comparison and a tendency to use comparisons as a means of criticising performance in Britain. Equally damning, many comparisons purport to refer to a 'British' policy model which bears little relation to reality. In this sense one of the arguments for more explicit national–regional comparison in the British Isles is in developing a more adequate picture of 'policy' for international comparison. Any comparison that refers to Britain without explicitly acknowledging the importance of regional differences is in danger of presenting a misleading picture of uniformity and coherence. Thus in housing (but not necessarily in other policy areas), acknowledgement of regional variation is a prerequisite for any effective summary of the situation and characteristics of 'housing in Britain'. In this sense the primary case for national–regional comparison in Britain is improving the existing view of policy. This does not imply that differences must be studied because they exist. But where the development and interpretation of evidence increasingly identifies local and regional factors as crucial both as the products of broader processes or as determinants of future situations we are unlikely to be able to take advantage of international comparative study without first of all coping with regional–national variations.

In this context two types of interpretation are immediately obvious. First that differences in the stock of housing, in tenure structure and in legislation governing housing in Scotland, Wales, Ireland and England indicate fundamentally different traditions and policy determinants. In this sense the case for comparison would be to explain differences in terms of economic, political and cultural factors that result in basic discontinuities. In such a model the differences between these regions/nations would serve to revise any unitary model of the welfare state and to offer more precise and specific models for comparison. Alternatively it could be that focusing interest on regional–national difference would draw attention to those social and economic processes that apply in each area but which result in spatial differences. For example, they would tend to lead us away from a view that legislation is the paramount element and that reference to legislation is adequate in summarising policy. The very fact of diversity in housing situations would require some examination of differences in legislation or in administrative and financial factors which might explain differences in the use of legislative power.

Attention might be drawn to the connections between housing and housing policy and political conflict or economic and employment circumstances. For example it might suggest that local political factors are more critical in determining policy output. With the exception of Northern Ireland where it has been accepted that the allocation and building of dwellings has been influenced by the geography of votes and where housing has been used as a reward for political loyalty, it is generally assumed that territorial defence is not an important factor in the political sphere. But a number of studies, and most recently Young and Kramer in London, suggest that such factors are more generally important.[2]

Similarly, the impact of economic and employment factors on new building, levels of investment in older housing, rates of house price inflation and consequent accumulation of wealth are much more crucial than is often recognised. In a situation where the public sector is increasingly developing into a housing sector for the poor, differential access to housing itself and to other resources through place of residence are increasingly likely to reflect market processes. In such a situation summaries of British housing policy would need to place a greater emphasis on those factors, including public policy, that enable or lead to differential accumulation of wealth through housing, and which as a result of that, affect access to a range of resources. In this respect the questions arising are not simply professional judgements about how far certain normative goals have been met but would draw attention to broader factors in the policy environment.

Housing policy is not only concerned with meeting housing need and a current demand for shelter. It is also concerned with influencing access to opportunities to save and accumulate wealth. The structure of housing subsidy and taxation provides different access to ownership of commodities which appreciate at different rates. While there are enormous variations in rates of appreciation of value of property within regions, the variation between regions has been a marked feature. Public policy is a major factor in the relative experience in this respect of owners and non-owners as well as of different groups of owners in different regions. An important feature of housing policy is its role in encouraging individual ownership and in facilitating accumulation of wealth. Analysis of the differential impact of policy would involve a regional–national dimension and explanation of this differential impact is an important aspect of the analysis of the impact of housing policy. Arguably it tells us more about public policy and the nature of public intervention in housing than a description of legislation or taxation treatment that does not refer to impact.

Essentially this argument is that without confronting national–regional differences there is a tendency to emphasise different aspects of the housing policy environment (and to refer to these in comparisons with other countries) than would apply if the comparisons are made. The tendency is to encourage concern with factors that local studies do not indicate to be important. The tendency is to encourage a focus on legislative development, on Westminster and Whitehall and on the stated aims of policy and conventional measures of policy effects. Local studies suggest not simply that Scotland or Northern Ireland is an exception to the rule but that it is the supposed rule which is wrong. The kinds of processes and circumstances that studies in, for example, London, Birmingham or Newcastle focus on are more compatible with studies of Glasgow or Belfast than with the bland centralist Westminster model. The lesson to be drawn from this is that understanding of key processes and developing a robust model of housing policy in Britain requires place specific local and regional case studies. This does not imply that key processes are spatial or local but that understanding broader social processes involves accounting for how observable spatial patterns of difference are produced.

Joan Higgins has argued that the selection of comparisons should depend on the aim of any comparison being made.[3] While this is indisputable, it is also clear that there are a wide range of aims that regional–national comparison can contribute to. There are certain clear advantages in comparisons where the range of sources of diversity is limited. There are areas of particular interest that could only be enlightened by international comparison. Most obviously, if the aim of comparison is to consider the housing problems or responses associated with particular political and economic systems or the operation and effectiveness of alternative courses of action or alternative modes of provision, the comparison must be with countries where such circumstances apply. But, especially in view of the methodological problems which may make other comparisons more problematic there is a case for considering how far there is any difference at regional–national level that can be relevant. Perhaps the most desirable approach to this is to consider specific proposals individually as they arise. Nevertheless there are current areas of policy interest where regional–national comparison is relevant and could possibly make as great a contribution as international comparison. Some examples of this are as follows:

1. The role of public housing and the significance for patterns of access to housing and other resources of a larger/smaller public sector (Scotland in particular);
2. Differential opportunities to accumulate wealth through housing;
3. Political and ideological influences on housing policy;
4. Links between housing and employment, migration and economic development;
5. The impact of different patterns of employment and unemployment on housing investment, mortgage foreclosure, mobility and choice;
6. Issues of territorial defence, discrimination and definitions of need;
7. Determinants of house prices and levels of investment in housing by all types of owners.

While it is desirable to start with aims, some indication of the range of aims for which regional–national comparisons are relevant can be drawn up by looking at sources of difference and variation between England, Scotland, Wales and Northern Ireland. While comparisons for the sake of comparison are undesirable, there is a need for periodic review to avoid any tendency to look only at yesterday's issues. In addition it is possible that the researcher seeking appropriate comparisons may neglect some out of ignorance. In the following list therefore the intention is to indicate some factors which are referred to as sources of variation in housing provision and hence types of issue which could be highlighted by national–regional comparison.

Formal explanations of variation

The legal framework

There are substantial differences in legislation between Scotland, England, Northern Ireland and Eire. In Northern Ireland it may be argued that legislation has lagged behind England and Scotland, but whatever view is taken some explanation of why these differences have arisen is relevant. In addition some of the differences could indicate lessons for policy. For example different approaches to homelessness or (in Scotland) legislation affecting older dwellings could indicate policy alternatives and offer the opportunity to learn from others' experience. How effective is the tolerable standard in Scotland in developing policies for sub-standard housing compared with the operation of English housing and public health legislation in similar circumstances? What are the consequences for similar groups of households being catered for under different legislation?

There are also important differences in the land tenure system in Scotland. Richardson, Vipond and Furbey have indicated how the system of feu duties in Edinburgh influenced the cost and pattern of building.[4] Scots law enabled multiple ownership of flats in tenements and with the system of feu duties combined to affect the housing situation.

The local administrative framework

There is greater potential to consider, explain and compare in this area. Northern Ireland's unified Housing Executive with limited local accountability, the three all-purpose authorities in Scotland, organisations such as the former Northern Ireland Housing Trust or the Scottish Special Housing Association are appropriate areas for study in the light of concerns about accountability, levels of responsibility, divided policy responsibility, 'non-political' housing administration and administrative reform. How do different administrative frameworks adapt to similar situations and how important are these factors in determining policy outputs and differences? As in other areas referred to here there is little available evidence on these issues.

The financial framework

Policy differences in this area are apparent and, for example, housing subsidy systems differ and have developed from different historic experiences. More important there is scope to consider how different policies will have different effects in the light of differences in incomes, rent and the economic environment. In this area the more interesting questions might be why policy has not diverged more substantially.

Central–local government relations

Issues such as housing subsidies and public expenditure control as well as Ministerial control and regulation draw attention to differences in central–local relations. Central–local relations in Northern Ireland prior to direct rule were very different from those that operated in Scotland or Wales. The experience of legislative devolution and administrative devolution has led to the adoption of different policies in different areas. There is clear potential to consider the reasons for these differences and their relative effects. Most recently, for example, different systems of housing planning (housing plans and housing investment programmes) have developed in each region and different approaches to the sale of council houses have been adopted. The differences involved are not usefully reduced to 'greater' or 'less' control but involve differences in structure, process and output which are not so simply summarised.

Wider considerations

There can be little dispute about the factors listed above as potential sources of variations in policy and as areas where study could both help to cast light on the nature of housing policy in Britain and provide some lessons for policy. The areas indicated above are not the only sources of variation, and it is important to consider other relationships which national–regional comparisons could cast light on.

Political and ideological factors

The most obvious political differences in the UK lie in Northern Ireland and in the sustained role of the nationalist parties in Wales and Scotland. But there are strong and independent traditions in the UK political parties in different regions of England as well as in Scotland and Wales. The Labour party in Scotland and Wales has strong independent traditions and different bases of support. How do these differences affect housing and other social policies? Attitudes to public housing and rents in Scotland or to leasehold enfranchisement in Wales reflect political and ideological factors as well as differences in 'need'. In addition the growth of housing pressure groups in England and Scotland has not been paralleled in Wales and Northern Ireland, and there is scope to consider the effect of such bodies and the voluntary sector generally.

Economic development

The nature of housing differences and problems is inextricably bound up with a pattern of economic development which is inherently uneven. Nineteenth century industrialisation, the decline of traditional industries and agriculture and the pattern of modern industrial investment have affected regions in different ways. The housing stock is of different ages and tenures and decays or is modernised and replaced at different rates, responding in large measure to economic changes and changes in market demand. Even public sector investment tends to follow or precede (as infrastructure in regional development policies) economic development. Flows of funds and of investment and disinvestment in housing associated with economic change outweigh those associated with direct public intervention in policy. In this sense some understanding of the relationship between housing and other investment or of the problems associated with economic change can be developed from national–regional study.

The housing market

The housing market remains predominantly a private market. Most housing is produced (except where direct labour is involved) by the private sector. The majority of housing (except in Scotland) is owned and controlled by private agencies. A wide range of institutions have developed around private housing. Processes of investment and decay in the stock and of access and mobility in housing crucially involve private individuals and agencies – landlords, building societies, valuers, estate agents, solicitors. These agencies are unlikely to operate in dramatically different ways in different nations/regions. Nevertheless, where regional housing stocks differ and house prices and incomes vary the operation of these agencies and the market as a whole determines patterns of access, choice and mobility.

The role of public housing

This naturally leads to a consideration of the nature of state intervention in housing. The direct provision of housing by local authorities, new town development corporations and housing associations has developed as a means of redistributing resources and access to housing. But levels of provision vary considerably as do the methods of allocation and control and the involvement of professionals and politicians. The types and ages of dwellings in the public sector also vary considerably. Crucial policy questions are involved in whether these differences have any substantial effect on households. But the related questions concern how far alternative or different means of intervention would achieve similar results, and national–regional comparisons can only cast light on this in the ways indicated above. The varied pressures on policy and practice at different levels of government do lead to significant policy differences incompatible with a monolithic view of the state or of government and the nature and role of public housing would appear to vary substantially at national–regional levels.

The output of policy

Many of the issues referred to above essentially concern the impact of various differences in and affecting policy. There are different dimensions of impact which could be considered and consideration of cost effectiveness and costs and benefits could be involved. But in every case some measurement of output is required. Conventional 'world series' comparison tends to rely on statistical comparisons and simple quantified measures. However the complaints levelled at this will stress the need for qualitative measures, for some indication of mobility and choice available to different groups of household (defined, say, according to household composition, relative positon in terms of income, social class or housing history). How do different economic, social or policy systems affect the housing opportunities of the elderly, the disabled, newly formed households, families with children, or single persons? How do the homeless or those with interrupted earnings, or those with low incomes fare under the different systems? At the present time comparative studies singularly fail to provide satisfactory evidence on these questions. The convinced supporter of the merits of public housing or owner-occupation in Britain is unlikely to be convinced that there are major lessons to be learned from international comparison unless evidence on access, mobility and choice is available. It is at this level that national–regional comparison can be most relevant. Rather than start with policy or institutional differences and attempt to evaluate (falling foul of all the intervening and contextual factors in such an evaluation), questions could be asked about choice and mobility or about how different social groups fare in different areas. While this could provide the basis of research on an international level (and has done so) methodological problems are enormous and explanations or policy conclusions less easy to develop. It might even be that national–regional comparisons of this type would contribute to developing methodology applicable in other comparisons. The nature of stratification in housing and the nature of housing ladders or filtering in the different regions are important questions for policy. In the light of tenure and other differences, do particular groups of households in Scotland, say, have a wider chance of obtaining a certain minimum standard of housing but have a more limited range of choice? In which situations are homeless families least well catered for and why? To what extent are low income households trapped in particular parts of the housing market and what are the implications of differences in the housing stock or tenure for this? We do not have examples of substantial attempts to deal with such questions and local case studies providing relevant data are not systematically compared. Such comparison need not amount to an attempt to say what system is best but would begin to identify crucial differences relevant to this.

The direct public provision of housing and means of access to it vary between areas. Although dramatic contrasts about public housing are more likely to emerge from the USA or Eastern Europe, public housing in Britain is nearer to a residual service in some areas than others and has different functions in territorial defence, social polarisation and residential segregation. While geographers have spent considerable time charting patterns of segregation the role of public policy in this has not been fully explored. Thus while patterns of segregation in Belfast are well established, the significance of housing market or public policy or income-occupation factors in this are not well researched. Similarly patterns of polarisation elsewhere have not received great attention. How far does public housing exacerbate or reduce polarisation and in what ways and under what circumstances? Issues of this type are conventional points of departure but have not been addressed by national–regional comparisons which could inform the debate.

For example, studies of filtering and household movement do lead to some tentative conclusions. One Northern Ireland study states:

> tenants in Northern Ireland are more likely to move to owner-occupation than is indicated in England. The size of the private rented stock and the relatively low price of houses for purchase would appear to be important here. Movement between tenures appears to be greater in Northern Ireland than in England. Thus for example movement by owner-occupiers to Housing Executive housing suggests a more 'open' housing market. Perhaps public sector housing is more acceptable in Northern Ireland because of its superior quality. It is not possible to draw firm conclusions on this question, but changes in rent control, housing finance and house prices are bound to have repercussions on mobility and opportunity and on household budgets. Such repercussions should be assessed prior to policy review.[5]

Since this report was written, policy on rent regulation in Northern Ireland has changed (it still differs from the rest of the UK), and house prices have risen dramatically, moving Northern Ireland from the position as the lowest priced region in the 1960 to the highest priced region other than South East (including Greater London) since between 1976 and 1979.[6] But what the significance of these changes have been and why they have occurred remain unexplored in spite of their potential significance.

While studies of filtering and movement or of institutions and patterns of use are relevant in this context direct analysis starting with the consumer is also appropriate. This is not met by general purpose housing surveys but requires analysis of how 'similar' households are affected by different traditions and regimes in housing – by different legislation and use of discretion over matters such as rents, action under public health and housing acts, rent control, housing allocation and transfers. How do single parent families fare in housing in Scotland, Wales, Northern Ireland and England? What are the crucial factors affecting different experience and how can they be remedied or modified? Such study implies a consideration not just of housing policy but of the relationship between housing and other policies. It would be equally useful to consider how client groups, defined because they have been in contact with 'social service' agencies, fare in different circumstances.

The case of homelessness[7]

The most obvious examples of how households' contacts with housing agencies differ involve reference to the homeless and (perhaps) housing applicants and tenants. The homeless are a particularly interesting group at the present time. The Housing (Homeless Persons) Act 1977 applies in Scotland, England and Wales. In Northern Ireland provision for the homeless is made under an emergency housing scheme while legal rights have not been revised in line with the rest of the UK. In Scotland, England and Wales, prior to the Housing (Homeless Persons) Act, responsibility for the homeless was placed, under the National Assistance Act 1948, with the local authority social services departments. Contrary to expectations in 1948 homelessness did not decline into a minimal problem and in spite of major expenditure on housing the numbers of homeless households increased considerably. In the 1960s increasing numbers and publicity drew attention to the failings of provision in practice. Communal facilities, segregation according to sex, restricted contact between husband and wife and arbitrary exclusion highlighted the reluctant, poor law attitude of authorities. Local authorities' provision for the homeless fell far short of that urged by central government or that enabled by legislative powers. In the 1960s a series of circulars urged co-operation to ensure that housing authorities took greater responsibility for housing the homeless, and while some local authorities did substantially change their approach, the homeless in some areas continued to rely on social services departments reluctant to accept responsibility.

The Housing (Homeless Persons) Act 1977 was the result of a private member's bill passed with government support. However, the bill as originally presented was based on a Department of Environment draft broadly designed to put into legislative effect a circular jointly issued by the DOE and the DHSS in 1974.[8] This transferred the duty to provide accommodation for the homeless to housing authorities and placed other duties in respect of homelessness on housing departments. As drafted by the DOE the bill had applied only to England and Wales. Its proposer, Stephen Ross, however, extended the bill to include Scotland after receiving presentations from several Scottish groups. The Secretary of State for Scotland had believed it not necessary to include Scotland and had been holding consultations to produce a code of practice to deal with homelessness on a voluntary basis. The legislation as it was passed did include Scotland although it took effect there four months later because it was considered that the Scottish local authorities (to whom the joint circular of 1974 had not applied) would take longer to prepare for implementation and only one housing authority had actually taken responsibility for the homeless prior to 1977. In addition to this difference the codes of guidance issued under section 12 of the Act differed. A joint DOE, DHSS and Welsh Office Code was produced for England and Wales while in Scotland guidance was provided in a circular[9] until a separate code was issued in September 1980.

Analysis of the impact of legislation on the homeless in Scotland, England, Wales and Northern Ireland would not however only refer to differences in legislation and codes of guidance. The Act gives enormous scope for varying interpretation and response is likely to be influenced by policial attitudes as well as the housing resources available and competing claims for them. Evidence on this is not currently available. However, research into homelessness could be concerned directly with this variation, with central-local government discussions on this, with the extent to which new legislation has changed policy and priorities, and its significance in different housing and political situations and for different groups. If the aim is to move beyond a picture of policy which refers principally to the formal policy arrangements and legislative details and to refer to practice, it may be relevant to consider how households declaring themselves homeless or potentially homeless fare in different parts of the UK. It may be that variation will be as great within, say, Scotland as between Scotland and Wales. Some evidence on the nature and types of differences which obtain and of any tendency to similarity within regions would be instructive and there are explanations which could be offered – ranging from the politician and professional to the attitudes of central departments, and political parties or the activities of pressure groups, to resources, the size and nature of the public housing stock and the other demands placed on it. An issue such as homelessness also draws in the need to examine the causes of homelessness and the activities of other agencies (and including social services) in dealing with households which are actually or potentially homeless.

Conclusions

What is suggested by the items above is that there are a variety of ways in which national-regional comparisons could contribute to understanding about the nature of housing policy and to the development of policy responses. It does not imply that such comparisons will necessarily yield more than international comparisons. But what is surprising is how underused the national-regional comparison is. Even for Scotland, which in housing has benefited from official and academic research interest, there is no systematic comparison and no attempt to evaluate or explain differences. In Northern Ireland, Wales and Eire the published literature is even more scarce.

In housing research, international comparative study has tended to run ahead of national–regional comparisons to an extent which strains the adequacy of our 'UK housing policy' picture and limits the lessons which can be learnt from such comparisons and to an extent which suggests that the choice of comparisons has not been based on considerations of the aims of comparison. Indeed, the initial aim has been too often to compare countries and their performance. Rather than for comparison to be a means to an end it has often been an end in itself. At this stage it is appropriate to reiterate the potential advantages of comparative study. Higgins suggests:

1. Considering whether problems of policy are peculiar to certain types of political and economic system or whether problems are inherent in the policies themselves;
2. Widening the range of policy options and knowledge of alternative courses of action;
3. Potential lesson learning;
4. Identifying and evaluating fashions in policy;
5. Identifying the social determinants of policy.[10]

There are examples throughout housing where national–regional comparisons can contribute in each of these ways. In addition we can add:

6. Developing a more robust and coherent picture of policy and of change, conflicts and inconsistencies within the UK which affect policy and the impact of policy.

There are inevitably a large number of reservations on the methodologies to be applied, the purpose of any comparison, the type of explanation which study precludes and the need for a framework of theories and hypotheses to structure comparison rather than compare simply because differences exist. Essentially this paper has argued that we cannot arrive at a view of what is generally true for housing policy in the UK without explicitly examining the national–regional demension. Existing evidence and theory suggests that the different economic circumstances, political traditions, administrative and legal frameworks and historical precedents which exist at the national–regional level must be understood and addressed before we can develop an adequate picture of housing policy at a general level. Without this the danger is that the view presented of housing policy does not exist anywhere in practice or is really, say, an English, Southern or Westminster interpretation of the welfare state. Because of the nature of differences there are also opportunities to examine policy alternatives and learn lessons and to avoid temptation in focusing on which system is best.

One of the interesting questions that emerges from any view that 'of course national–regional comparisons in housing are needed' is 'why have so few studies been carried out?' This raises questions about access to data and about funding and management of research and the predilection of government and other bodies. But it is also relevant to note the political sensitivity of the area. The regional issue and questions of devolution, independence, autonomy and levels of subsidy are sensitive politically. There will always be a fear that comparisons are ultimately likely to be used to criticise performance in a less than constructive manner. It may be therefore that the major funders of housing research – government departments – will never look on this area favourably and that initiatives will have to come from elsewhere.

Notes

1. For example, P. Wendt, *Housing Policy: The Search for Solutions*, University of California, 1963; G. Hallett, *Housing and Land Policies in West Germany and Britain*, London: Macmillan, 1978.
2. K. Young and J. Kramer, *Strategy and Conflict in Metropolitan Housing*, London: Heinemann, 1978.
3. Joan Higgins, *Approaches to Comparison in Social Policy*, (mimeo), paper presented to the SSRC workshop on the Comparative Study of the Social Sciences in the United Kingdom, May 1979.
4. H. W. Richardson, J. Vipond and R. Furbey, *Housing and Urban Spatial Structure: A Case Study*, Farnborough: Saxon House, 1975.
5. A. Murie *et al.*, 'New Building and Housing Need', in *Progress in Planning*, Vol. 6, Part 2, p. 155, Pergamon, 1976.
6. Building Societies Association, *Facts and Figures*, No. 29, January 1982.
7. For details on which this section draws heavily see Janet Richards, *The Housing (Homeless Persons) Act 1977: A Study in Policymaking*, Working Paper 22, School for Advanced Urban Studies, University of Bristol, 1981.
8. Circular DOE 18/74, DHSS 4/74, WO 34/74: *Homelessness.*
9. Circular SDD, 13/78.
10. Higgins, *Approaches to Comparison in Social Policy.*

11 Low Incomes in the Countries of the United Kingdom

Richard Berthoud

Other contributions to this book have considered variations between the four home countries in social policies and programmes. The focus, therefore, is on alternative responses to specific kinds of social 'need'. This chapter is concerned with rather an important need – people's need for an adequate income. There is, however, very little divergence indeed between the four home countries in public policy on incomes, whether this is direct intervention through taxation and cash benefits, global economic management, or governmental influence on industry and/or the labour market. In this all-important sector, policy usually applies nationwide, although many aspects of it are administered at the country level, at least in Northern Ireland. The aim of this chapter is, therefore, different from that of others; it will concentrate on variations in need in the four countries, rather than in the public response to need.

A number of indicators can be considered to show how far the residents of one of the constituent countries of the UK are better off or worse off than the residents of the others. The analysis is designed mainly to describe the differences between the countries, rather than to explain them, still less to suggest a solution. The chapter is intended to provide context for other, policy-oriented, chapters on the ground that it makes a deal of difference to an education programme, a health programmme or whatever, whether it is operating in a poor or a wealthy area.

The United Kingdom can be considered to consist of four countries from certain points of view: history, national loyalty, certain aspects of administration and ministerial responsibility, as well as the World Cup. For other administrative purposes, it is three countries (England and Wales being treated as a unit); or two (Great Britain counted as a unit); or a single country. An incidental pain in the neck for analysts of social and economic statistics, not least for the author of this chapter, is that the Government Statistical Service collectively appears to have no idea what country it is supposed to describe. It seems to be anyone's guess what area a particular set of figures will cover: how many of the countries will be included at all, how many will be combined for summary purposes, how many will be identifiable in detailed analysis. Ironically, Northern Ireland is least often included at all, England almost always; but if separate figures for each country are needed, they will almost always be available for Northern Ireland (if it was included at all), almost never for England as such.

Leaving aside the grouses of the researcher, a more substantial question is how variations between the four countries should be viewed. One way of looking at them, especially appropriate for those concerned with administrative variations, is simply the four-way comparison. From the point of view of statistical description, however, it should also be borne in mind that England, with 46.5 million population, comprises five-sixths of the United Kingdom. Scotland (5.2 million people), Wales (2.8 million) and Northern Ireland (1.5 million) are each so much smaller than England as a whole that they can be expected to diverge more from the national average.[1] They are more nearly equivalent in size to one of the Standard Regions in England; apart from the South East (16.9 million, including 6.9 million in Greater London) the English regions range in population from 6.5 million (North West) to 1.9 million (East Anglia). Although the focus in this chapter will be on the four home countries, the range of variation between the regions of England will also be quoted, to indicate whether the three smaller countries are in a class of their own, or within the normal span of inter-regional differences.

Population structure

Wherever they live in the UK, people participate in approximately the same social and economic system, and are subject to the same taxes and benefits. It is therefore appropriate to begin the examination of income needs by considering the structure of the home countries' populations. If there are certain types of family which are generally at risk of poverty – wherever they live – then an unusually large population of such families in any of the home countries would suggest a high level of income need, quite independent of any local economic factors.

Table 11.1 shows the relative risk of poverty according to families' basic demographic and economic structure. The figures, derived from the General Household Survey[2] cover Great Britain only, but would certainly look almost identical if the whole of the UK were included. Old people, especially lone old women, have an above-average risk of poverty, and account for well over half of all poor families. The greatest risk of poverty, however, is experienced by lone parents. Moreover (not shown in the table) this group is unique in the proportion of its members who fall a long way below the conventional poverty line.[3] A third concentration of poverty is found among families with four or more children. The second half of Table 11.1 largely reflects the first, showing, as one would expect, that poverty is closely related to economic activity. The economically inactive consist mainly of pensioners but also include the disabled and a proportion of lone parents. (The unemployed, to be considered later in this chapter, are defined as economically active, their 'activity' consisting of looking for, and being available to accept, a job.)

Thus there will tend to be a lot of poverty in any part of the country where elderly or other economically inactive people are common or where there are many lone parents or large families. There are only two substantial sources of data on household structures which cover the whole country, including Northern Ireland, and neither is entirely satisfactory. One is the Census,[4] which, although it usually presents data for different home countries in separate volumes, is conducted on the same basis throughout the Kingdom. On the other hand, we are at the time of writing (July 1982), in the worst of the trough of the Census's ten-year cycle – the figures now available are eleven years out of date, but because of the enormous volume of data to be processed, last year's detailed statistics have not yet been issued.

An attractive alternative source of data is the Family Expenditure Survey covering a sample of about 7000 households annually, throughout the United Kingdom.[5] Not only does this survey include Northern Ireland as well as Great Britain; a separate report on the Province is also published which can provide some figures on a larger sample than is incorporated in the overall results.[6] The FES is often used to provide demographic data on a regional basis. The interviews for the survey are, however, both voluntary and very complex. The participation rate is usually about 70%. This would not matter much if it could be shown that low response had not biased the results one way or another. However, as far as Northern Ireland specifically is concerned, there is a demonstrable bias. As Table 11.2 shows, a surprisingly large proportion of the households cooperating about the time of the 1971 Census contained elderly/economically inactive people. It looks like the strength of this bias has increased over the 1970s so that Northern Ireland, actually with a relatively small elderly population, appears from the FES to have an exceptionally high proportion in this age group. One may guess that this bias derives from progressive withdrawal of cooperation among certain types of younger family in Northern Ireland, as a result of the political problems of the Province. In 1979, only just over half (53%) of the heads of household who agreed to take part in the survey in Northern Ireland were categorised as economically active.[7] The true figure should probably exceed 70%. It appears, however, that the 1980

Table 11.1 **Analysis of poverty according to family type and economic activity (%)**

	Married couples				*Non-married adults*				*All families*
	Pensionable age	*Others without children*	*With children 1–3*	*With children 4 or more*	*Pensionable age man*	*Pensionable age woman*	*Others without children*	*With children*	
Risk of poverty	20	3	5	25	26	38	6	41	13
Share of poverty	13	4	10	3	6	44	10	9	100
	Both economically active	*One active*	*Neither active*			*Active*	*Inactive*		
Risk of poverty	1	8	27			6	41		13
Share of poverty	3	13	14			10	59		100

Source: Richard Berthoud and Joan C. Brown, *Poverty and the Development of Anti-Poverty Policy in the UK*, London: Heinemann/PSI, 1981. Derived from the 1975 General Household Survey.

Note: 'In poverty' is defined as an annual equivalent income lower than the adult long-term rate of Supplementary Benefit.

survey was somewhat less affected by this bias than its immediate predecessor.

Table 11.2 Indicators of elderly/economically inactive households in the population (%)

	England	*Wales*	*Scotland*	*Northern Ireland*	*United Kingdom*
Proportion of households containing no economically active person					
1971 Census	21	23	20	17	20
1971/72 FES	20	23	21	23	19
1979/80 FES	25	29	23	29	25
Proportion of individuals in private households aged 65 or more					
1971 Census	12.9	13.5	11.9	10.4	12.7
1971/72 FES	11.6	11.7	11.4	11.8	11.6
1980 Population estimates	15.1	15.3	14.0	11.7	14.8
1979/80 FES	13.8	15.1	11.1	15.0	13.6

Sources: *Census 1971; Family Expenditure Survey; Regional Trends*
Note: The population estimates in the penultimate line of the table include people not in private households, and therefore naturally give a higher proportion of old people than would truly reflect the population in private households – the basis for the other three sets of figures. Note that the FES-based estimates are included here only to indicate the bias in FES data, as discussed in text.

In practice, therefore, it will be safer to use the 1971 Census to indicate the extent of any inter-country variation in household structures, using other data as are available to suggest whether the picture has changed much since then. At the level of generality with which we are concerned, the four countries are, not surprisingly, essentially similar. Northern Ireland, physically more separate and incorporating some more diverse cultural patterns than the other three countries, stands out somewhat in the youth of its population: it has a relatively substantial number of large families, and rather a small number, as already noted, of households dependent on elderly and economically inactive people. Northern Ireland also appeared to have relatively the largest number of one-parent families in 1971, although more recent data derived from payments of Lone Parent Benefit do not suggest that the Province is still the leader in this respect. Northern Ireland can be expected to exhibit relatively little pensioner poverty, but a large element of family poverty, compared with the rest of the United Kingdom.

Scotland's demographic structure has special features similar to that of Northern Ireland, but they are less notable. There are slightly fewer pensioner households in Scotland than in England and Wales, rather

Table 11.3 Indicators of the number of large families in the population (%)

	England	*Wales*	*Scotland*	*Northern Ireland*	*United Kingdom*
Households with 4 or more children, 1971					
as a proportion of all households	3.3	3.3	4.7	10.1	3.6
as a proportion of households with any children	8.3	8.7	11.4	21.3	9.4
Families receiving child benefit for 4 or more children, 1980, as a proportion of all CB families	4.4	4.3	4.8	13.8	4.7

Sources: *Census 1971; Social Security Statistics; Department of Health and Social Services – NI*, private communication.

Table 11.4 Indicators of the number of lone parent families in the population (%)

	England	*Wales*	*Scotland*	*Northern Ireland*	*United Kingdom*
Households containing children with one adult, 1971					
as a proportion of all households	1.4	1.3	1.5	1.8	1.4
as a proportion of households with any children	3.7	3.2	3.7	3.9	3.7
Families receiving child benefit increase, 1980					
as a proportion of all CB families	6.1	5.5	6.5	5.5	6.1

Sources: As Table 11.3.
Note: Child Benefit Increase is now known as Lone Parent Benefit. The use of this benefit to estimate the number of lone parents is not ideal, as the take-up rate is less than 100%.

more large families and one-parent families. Wales, however, shows the opposite characteristics, with marginally the largest elderly population and relatively small numbers of families at risk of poverty. Nevertheless, the overall conclusion must be that England, Wales and Scotland have population structures which would lead one to expect roughly the same level of poverty in each country; Northern Ireland shows differences in its population which might well affect the structure of its poverty, although by balancing one feature against the other one might expect the total proportion of households on low incomes to be the same in Northern Ireland as elsewhere.

Low incomes

There are two approaches to the geographical assessment of income needs. One is to enquire whether the total pool of income in an area is adequate for the number of people living there. The other approach is to look at individual households in the area to see how many lack an adequate income. In this analysis, however, the question of what level of income is adequate will not be tackled directly; it will be assumed that a country has a relative need if its income level is lower than that of the other home countries.

The obvious source of data on household incomes is, of course, the *Family Expenditure Survey*. However, it has been shown above that this survey contains a serious bias, specifically in Northern Ireland, which makes an inter-country comparison rather risky. If there are proportionately too many elderly/economically inactive households in the FES sample in Northern Ireland, that will tend to understate income levels or overstate the amount of poverty. On the other hand there is some evidence that the number of large families is also under-represented in the FES Northern Ireland sample, and this may redress the balance somewhat when the sample as a whole is being considered. Fortunately, it is possible to compare the FES with other sources. Each of these has drawbacks of its own, but if all tell a similar story, greater trust can be placed in the conclusions.

Considering the total income pool, the two sources shown in the first half of Table 11.5 are not nearly as comparable as they appear. Both the FES and the Central Statistical Office's national accounts have their own drawbacks, and differ on so many points of detail that direct comparison between them is extremely hazardous. But the consistency between the two sources in the comparison between the four home countries is impressive. The main difference between the two is that the FES places Scotland and Wales about level, while the CSO figures give Scotland a clear edge.

Turning to the identification of individual households with low incomes, the FES is more easily compared with the results of Townsend's 1968 survey of *Poverty in the United Kingdom.*[8] The Royal Commission on the Distribution of Incomes and Wealth[9] analysed the 1976 FES on an 'equivalent income' basis which is similar, though not identical, to Townsend's use of Supplementary Benefit scale rates to compare households with different needs. The Royal Commission chose to analyse the

Table 11.5 Indicators of household incomes

	England			Wales	Scotland	Northern Ireland	United Kingdom
	Average	*Best*	*Worst*				
Average income per head per week (£)							
Personal disposable income, National Accounts, 1980	56.1	62.0 (SE)	50.9 (N)	50.7	53.4	44.4	55.3
Gross normal income, Family Expenditure Survey, 1979/80	50.5	57.4 (SE)	44.1 (YH)	45.4	45.7	38.3	49.5
Proportion with low incomes (%)							
Households below national lower quartile, of equivalent income, FES 1976	24	21 (EM)	29 (N)	31	28	38	25
Individuals in households below 140% of SB rate, Townsend, 1968	27[a]	24 (SE)	34 (NW)	n.a.	29	44	28

Sources: Line 1 – *Regional Trends*;
Line 2 – *Family Expenditure Survey*;
Line 3 – Royal Commission on the Distribution of Incomes and Wealth, *Report no. 6, Lower Incomes*, London: HMSO, 1978;
Line 4 – Peter Townsend, *Poverty in the United Kingdom*. Harmondsworth, Penguin, 1979.

Note: [a]England and Wales.

lowest quarter of all households; Townsend's cut-off point happened to cover 28% of individuals. Townsend's survey had a much higher response rate than the FES (though he did not quote a separate response rate for Northern Ireland). On the other hand, the FES has a much larger sample, and Townsend's Northern Ireland sample of three electoral wards can scarcely be considered to represent the whole of the Province reliably. But, in spite of these differences, the two sources are at least consistent in showing the same inter-country variations in the relative number of low income households, parallel with the variations also observed in the size of the total income pool.

It may be concluded, therefore, that Scottish households tend to have somewhat lower incomes in relation to their needs than English households; that Welsh households are slightly worse off than Scottish; but that Northern Irish households have, on the whole, lower incomes than those in any of the constituent parts of Great Britain.

These conclusions need to be seen in two important perspectives. First, consider each of the three smaller countries as 'regions' of the United Kingdom, to be compared with the regions of England which are more nearly equivalent in size. Table 11.5 shows, for each measure of low income, the best and worst of the English regions. Northern Ireland stands, in all four cases, well outside the range of regional variation within England. Scotland and Wales, on the other hand, appear to lie on the fringe of the variations observed within England. While they are clearly poorer – much poorer – than some regions of England, they are little poorer, sometimes less poor, than others. As a general rule, London and/or the South-East of England seem to have the highest incomes. The regions furthest from London, especially the Northern and North-Western regions, tend to show the lowest incomes. In that context, Scotland and Wales could be seen as the extremities of a northern and western axis of low incomes. If so, their poverty, relative to the southern and eastern corner of Great Britain, may stem from their geographical position, rather than specifically from any constitutional, racial or other characteristic that distinguishes them from England.

Northern Ireland, on the other hand, appears to occupy an income position outside the normal range of regional variation. It is, of course, the extreme north-western region of the Kingdom. But if income levels were plotted in relation to north-westerly mileages, the plot might have to be extended almost to Iceland to find a position whose expected income level was as low as that observed in Ulster.

However, even the gap between Northern Ireland and the best off regions of Great Britain may appear small when seen in its widest perspective. While one region may have a lower average income, or a larger proportion of low income households, than another, it is perfectly clear that there are many prosperous people in the one, and many poor in the other. That is, the range of variation between regions is tiny in comparison with the range of variation between households. One crude estimate has suggested that there is forty times as much inequality between households as between regions.[10] That estimate relates to England and Wales, but it is clear that even if the outlying home countries were included in the calculation, a household's income would be seen to depend far more on its own position up the local ladder, than on the local ladder's position in the national scale.

Nevertheless, the statistics agree that Scotland and Wales are somewhat deprived of income in comparison with much of England, and Northern Ireland is quite severely deprived. Peter Townsend's graphic description of the appearance of poverty on his first visit to Northern Ireland in 1968 emphasised the out-of-dateness of what he saw: '. . . scenes which seemed to belong more to the 1930s – of red-haired boys using scales on a cart drawn by an emaciated pony to sell coal by the pound. . . .'[11] Indeed, anachronism may be considered central to the concept of relative poverty in an age of increasing prosperity. Conditions are now described as 'poor' which were quite normal thirty years ago. Think of running hot water, indoor WCs, televisions, adequate heating and so on, all considered luxuries within living memory, but so essential now that the lack of them represents deprivation. In that case, an illustration of an area's poverty might be an estimate of how far it is behind the times. In the housing field, Northern Ireland is known to lag far behind Great Britain, but this is because of historical problems of housing policy, rather than a direct reflection of low incomes.[12] But the Family Expenditure Survey suggests that the penetration of many consumer durables has lagged several years behind in Northern Ireland, compared with Great Britain (Table 11.6), even though Townsend's implicit suggestion that Ulster is thirty years behind the times may be something of an exaggeration.

Table 11.6 Penetration of consumer durables (%)

	United Kingdom		*England*	*Wales*	*Scotland*	*Northern Ireland*
	1969/70	*1979/80*	*1979/80*	*1979/80*	*1979/80*	*1979/80*
Cars	51	59	60	61	49	52
Central heating	27	57	59	55	49	33
Washing machine	64	78	77	81	82	60
Refrigerator	63	94	99	94	93	80
Television	91	96	96	98	97	91
Telephone	34	69	71	58	70	49

Source: *Family Expenditure Survey.*

Low pay

The so-called 'New' Earnings Survey, which has been carried out annually since 1970, is published separately for Great Britain and for Northern Ireland.[13] Indeed, few analysts of the British data are aware that the Northern Ireland survey exists. The enquiry is a survey among employers of PAYE participants, and therefore excludes the self-employed. All the figures quoted here refer to full-time adult employees.

The most recent data suggest a pattern of male earnings rather similar to the pattern of household incomes just discussed. Scotland and Wales have slightly lower average wages, and slightly higher proportions of men on low pay, than England, but are not dissimilar to the lower paid regions of England. Men in Northern Ireland, on the other hand, average 8% below the English figure, and this is most noticeable at the lower end of the distribution: proportionately twice as many Ulster men as Englishmen earned wages below £75 in 1981, a wage which, depending on their family commitments, might leave them in poverty even with a permanent full-time job. Those family commitments may be considerable: it should be remembered that there is an exceptional number of large families in Northern Ireland, and it will be seen below that there are relatively few working mothers. The problem of low pay is therefore of critical importance to the question of family poverty in the Province. It should, however, be noted that there was some improvement in Northern Ireland men's earnings over the 1970s, relative to wages available in Great Britain.

Women's earnings have always been substantially lower than men's, all over the country, although equal pay and equal opportunities legislation have led to some reduction in the gap over the 1970s. At both ends of the decade Englishwomen were less likely to be low-paid than those in the other three countries. But the gap between the home countries is much narrower for women's earnings than for men'; indeed, there are some regions within England that are somewhat worse off than any of the three small countries in this respect, and, for once, Northern Ireland does not seem in a class of its own.

Unemployment

Households dependent on the earnings of a single breadwinner face, of course, a severe risk of poverty if that person is unemployed for any length of time. Such poverty may be said to be a conscious consequence of government policy, in that the supplementary benefit rate for the unemployed remains below the poverty line implied by the long-term scale, however long the claimant remains out of work.

Table 11.7 Indicators of earnings

	England			Wales	Scotland	Northern Ireland	United Kingdom
	Average	Best	Worst				
Men							
Average earnings (£)							
1971	33.1	35.8 (SE)	30.1 (EA)	31.8	31.3	28.8	32.8
1981	141	152 (SE)	132 (WM)	133	140	130	140
Proportion low paid (%)							
1971 (below £19)	7.9[a]	n.a	n.a.	n.a.	n.a.	17.9	8.1
1981 (below £75)	5.3	4.1 (SE)	7.4 (SW)	6.9	5.9	10.9	5.5
Women							
Average earnings (£)							
1971	18.4	20.1 (SE)	16.7 (YH)	17.8	17.4	16.7	18.3
1981	92	100 (SE)	85 (EM)	88	87	89	91
Proportion low paid (%)							
1971 (below £19)	71[a]	n.a.	n.a.	n.a	n.a.	74	71
1981 (below £75)	38	28 (SE)	48 (YH)	44	46	44	39

Sources: *Northern Ireland New Earnings Survey.*
Note: [a]Great Britain.

Over most of the post-war period, however, unemployment has contributed relatively small numbers to the total of UK poverty. Even as late as 1975, when the number of registered unemployed had reached nearly a million, only about one in ten poor households could blame unemployment;[14] the great majority of the poor took no part at all in the labour market. But recent trends in unemployment – especially in long-term unemployment – and in social security measures for the unemployed, suggest that the numbers of families in poverty through unemployment will have increased dramatically.

Because of recent public interest in unemployment rates, and because the Department of Employment publishes monthly statistics for the whole of the UK and for each region, the relative position of the home countries is reasonably well known.[15] As with incomes and earnings, Wales and Scotland have persistently been found to suffer unemployment at about the level of the worst-hit regions of England, and therefore have suffered more than the average for England as a whole. But, again, Northern Ireland fares substantially worse than any other region in the Kingdom, with nearly one in five of its workers unemployed. A focus on the most serious cases accentuates this disparity: in Northern Ireland, one male worker in ten has been out of work for more than a year; in Wales and Scotland, one in fifteen; in England, on average, one in twenty-one, and in the South East, one in thirty-four.

But, while unemployment rates in Northern Ireland are at a post-war high, it would be a mistake to ascribe this either specifically to the current nationwide crisis, or to the detrimental effects of over a decade of violence on the local economy. The Province suffered unemployment throughout the 1950s and 1960s at levels which have been considered to represent a crisis now that they have penetrated to England. The figures in Table 11.8 show that Northern Ireland's unemployment rate 'only' trebled between 1950 and 1982; in England, it multiplied nearly ten-fold.

One of the known deficiencies of the statistics on the registered unemployed is that they understate unemployment among married women, who, if they do not qualify for any benefit, may not register at Jobcentres while they are looking for work.[16] Figures on the size of this underestimate, derived from the *General Household Survey*, cover Great Britain, and therefore cannot be used for a full inter-country comparison. A longer-term consequence of acute scarcity of work might be that some married women who found no opportunity would cease to consider themselves as potential employees. In statistical terms they would become economically inactive, but in practice this may be seen as a form of unemployment. Married women in Northern Ireland might be expected to have an exceptionally strong motive to take paid work, since, as has been said, their husbands suffer below average pay and have an exceptional

Table 11.8 **Indicators of unemployment (%)**

	England			*Wales*	*Scotland*	*Northern Ireland*	*United Kingdom*
	Average	*Best*	*Worst*				
Annual averages							
1950	1.2	–	–	3.7	3.1	5.8	1.6
1960	1.3	–	–	2.7	3.6	6.7	1.7
1970	2.3	–	–	3.8	4.2	6.8	2.6
1980	6.8	–	–	10.3	10.0	13.7	7.4
January 1982							
Overall rate	12.0	9.2 (SE)	16.4 (N)	16.2	15.3	19.7	12.7
Males unemployed over one year	4.7	2.9 (SE)	7.4 (N)	6.7	6.1	10.4	5.0

Sources: *Abstract of Historical Labour Statistics, 1886 to 1968; Department of Employment Gazette.*

risk of unemployment. It has also been seen that many Northern Ireland mothers have large families: this constitutes both an incentive to take employment (children require food and clothing) and a disincentive (they need care and attention). Whatever the motivation, the unemployment figures indicate severe restrictions on job opportunities, and it seems clear that economic activity rates among married women are substantially lower in Northern Ireland than in Great Britain. Married women in Wales also show relatively low economic activity rates, and this may contribute to the Principality's position as one of the poorest regions on the mainland.

Table 11.9 Indicators of economic activity among married women (%)

	England	*Wales*	*Scotland*	*Northern Ireland*	*United Kingdom*
1971 census: married women aged 21–44	47	40	43	33	46
1979/80 FES: married women with children	62	51	60	50	61

Sources: *Census 1971; Family Expenditure Survey.*

Social assistance

Apart from benefits which are available at local authorities' discretion, the social security system applies uniformly across Great Britain, and is almost identical in Northern Ireland. But if the rules are universal, their effect can vary. The intention here is to compare the incidence of the two principal government instruments for the relief of poverty among those out of work and in work respectively.

Supplementary benefit is available to those not in work, and consists essentially of an allowance 'topping up' any other benefit or source of income to a prescribed minimum level, determined in accordance with one of two 'scale rates'. The higher or long-term rate is applied to pensioners (and their wives), and also to other claimants (and their wives) after a year on the basic rate. But claimants required to register for employment are not allowed to claim at the long-term rate, however long they have been out of work. Nor is there a higher rate available to assess the long-term needs of children, whatever their parents' status. All claimants on supplementary benefit are forced to live on very low incomes; those unemployed, or with children, or both, suffer a standard of living even lower than that of other claimants. The scheme will therefore be weakest in areas where it has to support many unemployed and/or children. It will come as no surprise, following the findings of earlier

Table 11.10 Social assistance (%)

	England	Wales	Scotland	Northern Ireland	United Kingdom
Supplementary Benefit					
Pensioner claimants: ratio to population aged 65+	21	22	20	31	21
Unemployed claimants as proportion of registered unemployed	50	50	45	60	50
Unemployed as proportion of claimants	26	30	34	36	28
Ratio of dependants per claimant	0.53[a]	n.a.	n.a.	0.79	0.54
Family Income Supplement					
Two-parent families	0.6	1.1	0.7	3.5	0.7
One-parent families	11.5	11.0	18.0	9.5	12.1

Sources: *Social Security Statistics*; *Department of Health and Social Services – NI.*
Note: [a]Great Britain. All figures relate to 1980.

sections of this chapter, that Northern Ireland has more SB claimants per head of population, more unemployed claimants and more claimants with children, than any other part of the United Kingdom. In other words, the supplementary benefit scheme's weaknesses are clearest exactly where the need of the population is strongest.

The family income supplement (FIS) was introduced in 1971 to provide a means-tested social assistance to families bringing up children on low wages. It makes up half the difference between the parents' earnings and a 'prescribed amount'. The scheme is much used by lone mothers, partly because they experience the exceptionally low female wage rates shown in Table 11.7 above, partly because they work part-time, and FIS has been especially adapted to include part-time working lone parents. Lone parents in Scotland have a higher rate of partial dependance on FIS than their counterparts elsewhere. In Great Britain, only a tiny proportion of two-parent families augment their income with FIS, but in Northern Ireland it is far more common among two-parent families. The reasons for this will by now be clear: on average in Northern Ireland, families have more children to support, have lower wages available to the breadwinner and a more limited opportunity to work for the breadwinner's spouse. The number of two-parent families on FIS in Northern Ireland is the clearest illustration of family poverty there.

Government policy

It is clear from the whole of the evidence quoted in this chapter that there is fairly substantial variation in income levels between the countries of the United Kingdom. This is not at all surprising – the three other large countries in the EEC all show internal variations in these types of measure on at least the scale observed here. Regional variation within each country may also be seen as part of diversity between regions across Europe. Indeed, in so far as it is legitimate to make comparisons across national boundaries, it can be noted that the Republic of Ireland experiences lower incomes and higher unemployment than even the worst region of the United Kingdom.[17] Northern Ireland's position may perhaps be explained in terms of its links with both economic networks.

But it is clearly one of the responsibilities of the United Kingdom government to identify need wherever it may be, and to take steps to eliminate inequalities. In its direct income support measures this is exactly what happens: taxes and benefits are virtually identical throughout the Kingdom. The income support network is impartial between regions, although, as has been noted, some of its shortcomings are more glaring in some areas than in others.

Given that the public sector makes up something like half of the national economy, a second form of government intervention lies simply in local public expenditure. This has an important general economic effect in addition to its various direct objectives of provide housing, education and so on. Table 11.11 shows that, as far as that proportion of public expenditure that can be attributed to one or other of the home countries is concerned, Wales and Scotland receive slightly more, in relation to their population size, than England does. Northern Ireland heads the table for receipt of public money, receiving about £8 for every £5 paid out in England.

Table 11.11 Indicators of government support (£ per annum)

	England	*Wales*	*Scotland*	*Northern Ireland*	*United Kingdom*
Expenditure per head 1980/81					
Economic support[a]					
Regional/industrial support	8	42	30	143	15
Labour market	30	46	34	43	32
Other	27	67	75	126	36
Other expenditure	1274	1604	1557	1634	1326
Expenditure on economic support[a] per unemployed worker	2200	3887	3172	6117	2599

Sources: *Regional Trends*; *Estimates of Services under the Government of Northern Ireland; The Government's Expenditure Plans.*

Note: [a]'Economic support' is used here to cover items headed 'industry, energy trade and employment,' and 'agriculture, fisheries, food and forestry'.

This bias in favour of the more needy home countries tends to apply across most fields of public service, including for instance, health and social services as well as social security, roads as well as law and order.[18] In most fields, the bias is rather slight, but it is substantial in those areas of government policy that are directly concerned with stimulation of the economy and of employment. One of the longest running programmes in this field is, of course, the regional development policy. Northern Ireland as a whole, and large areas of Wales and Scotland, qualify for help under this programme. It is generally believed at least to have helped prevent regional inequalities deteriorating further.[19] While there may be doubts as to whether the amount of money available is adequate, it is clear that much of it has been directed to those of the home countries whose need was greatest (Table 11.11).

A second type of programme consists of assistance to individual workers in the form of training, work experience, employment subsidy and so on. Such schemes have proliferated in the 1970s. Inter-country comparison of the scale of public labour market activities is hampered by their variety – it is not just a question of adding numbers together – and by the fact that they are administered independently in Northern Ireland. Total expenditure on these programmes (in relation to population size) was considerably higher in Wales and Northern Ireland than in England and Scotland.

Third, Table 11.11 confirms that other types of expenditure under industrial, employment, agricultural and similar headings is also tipped substantially towards Scotland and Wales, and heavily towards Northern Ireland. Indeed, the figures at the foot of the table suggest that these public efforts to stimulate the economy and reduce unemployment are very heavily concentrated in the areas where unemployment is worst.

Conclusion

It is not within the scope of this chapter to probe deeper into the structure of regional economies to explain why one part of the United Kingdom should suffer lower incomes than another. Low incomes tend to be suffered by certain types of household wherever they live, and geographical variations in 'need' may be explained partly in terms of the distribution of retired people, of lone parents, of the disabled and of large families. But there are clear economic variations as measured by the national accounts, by surveys, by wage rates and by unemployment rates. Governments have made efforts to redress these imbalances, although it is arguable either that these efforts have been insufficient to the task, or that they have been countered by other national policies that tend to concentrate wealth in the south-eastern corner of England.

On the mainland of Great Britain, both Wales and Scotland show more evidence of low incomes than does England as a whole. But if they are compared with English regions of a similar size, then the two smaller countries can be seen to be rather similar to other relatively poor areas remote from London. It is possible to see Welsh and Scottish problems as a symptom of general inequality across Britain; if so, a solution may be sought in an overall regional policy, as much as in specific programmes for the Celtic fringe. Poverty in Northern Ireland is, however, much more severe, and does seem to constitute a special problem in its own right, over and above a general regional economic imbalance.

This is by no means to say that poverty is confined to that Province. There are poor towns even in relatively prosperous England, poor districts even in wealthy cities, and, of course, poor people everywhere. Nor are wages in Northern Ireland as low in relation to Britain as they used to be. Poverty in Ulster is brewed from unemployment, low pay, and a social security network which is deficient, especially in its provisions for children. This is exactly the same recipe as applies in England, Wales and Scotland. An antidote is required at national level, but the adverse economic position of the regions, and especially of Northern Ireland, will need to be tackled at the same time.

Notes

1. Central Statistical Office *Regional Trends*, London: HMSO, annual.
2. Office of Population Censuses and Surveys, *General Household Survey*, London: HMSO, annual.
3. Richard Berthoud and Joan C. Brown, *Poverty and the Development of Anti-Poverty Policy in the UK*, London: Heinemann/PSI, 1981.
4. Office of Population Censuses and Surveys, *Census 1971*, London: HMSO, 1971 onwards. See also General Register Offices – Scotland and Northern Ireland.
5. Department of Employment, *Family Expenditure Survey*, London: HMSO, annual.
6. Department of Finance – NI, *Northern Ireland Family Expenditure Survey*, Belfast: HMSO, annual.
7. *Northern Ireland Family Expenditure Survey*.
8. Peter Townsend, *Poverty in the United Kingdom*, Harmondsworth: Penguin, 1979.
9. Royal Commission on the Distribution of Incomes and Wealth, Report no. 6, *Lower Incomes*, London: HMSO, 1978.
10. Richard Berthoud, 'Where are London's poor?', *Greater London Intelligence Quarterly*, 1976.
11. *Poverty in the United Kingdom*, p. 558.
12. See, for example, Eileen Evason, *Poverty, the Facts in Northern Ireland*, Child Poverty Action Group, 1976.
13. Department of Employment, *New Earnings Survey*, London: HMSO, annual; Department of Manpower Services – NI, *Northern Ireland New Earnings Survey*, Belfast: annual.
14. Berthoud and Brown, *Poverty and the Development of Anti-Poverty Policy in the UK*.
15. *Department of Employment Gazette*, London: HMSO, monthly.
16. W. W. Daniel, *The Nature of Current Unemployment*, British North American Research Association, 1981.
17. See, for example, *Regional Trends*.
18. See *Regional Trends*.
19. Organisation of Economic Cooperation and Development, *Regional Policies, the Current Outlook*, Paris: 1977.

PART FOUR
Bibliographical Essay

12 Comparing areas: a review and bibliography of literature on the health and personal social services in which there are elements of comparison between areas of the United Kingdom

Gillian Stewart

Literature review

It is often claimed that social administration is an eclectic subject, drawing its theoretical bases and methods of analysis from other disciplines.[1] Such a claim of eclecticism gains some credibility from examination of the published literature on the health and personal social services in which there are elements of comparison between areas of the UK. The collection of literature here presented is fragmented, showing little evidence of cohesiveness nor of mutual awareness between the different authors, outside discrete specialisms. It would be difficult to regard this published literature as representing a coherent and established discipline of comparative study of the social services within the UK. Nevertheless, and although this is a preliminary bibliography, it is possible to suggest some general trends.

Academic traditions to which some authors in this bibliography belong include:

1. *Human geography*, involving areal analysis and spatial aspects of the incidence of social problems or the use of social services among a given population (Warnes 1982, ref. 25);
2. *Epidemiology*, when a geographical dimension is identified in the incidence of illness;
3. *Welfare microeconomics*, where the principles and logistics of resource allocation and the pattern of demand for services, contain a geographically comparative element;
4. *Anthropology*, through the study of neighbourhoods (Warren 1981, ref. 28);
5. *Sociology of community*, including potentially relevant research not here listed (a search among the 'community studies' of the 1950s and early 1960s might prove fruitful).

Political analysis is a perspective not normally adopted in comparative research within the UK, unlike internationally comparative studies.[2]

Domestic comparative studies have been concerned with administrative aspects of the social services, rather than with ideology and analysing the formation of social policies. Not surprisingly, perhaps, as broad policy directions for local personal social services are supposed to be prescribed by central government, and the health service is even more centralised. Local administrative interpretations of nationally defined policies are the subject of comparisons. In this respect, domestic comparative studies fall within the empirical and prescriptive Fabian mainstream of social administration as an academic subject.[3]

A central concept in domestic comparative social administration is that of 'territorial (in)justice', developed principally by Bleddyn Davies (ref. 79). Government recognition of injustice derived from geographical variation in services, was expressed in the 1976 DHSS Consultative Document:

> There is . . . a need progressively to remedy the large variations in standards between different regions, areas, and districts . . . . How far these variations reflect differences in need is not known for certain, but there are clearly major inequities in the distribution of services which must be corrected.[4]

Complex deprivation indicators and methods of measuring and comparing 'need' have been developed (Holterman 1975, ref. 58). A new and substantial body of literature is concerned with area treatment programmes based on principles of positive discrimination. Though not as coherent as the latter, another body of literature presents inter-authority comparisons of provision of, and access to, social services (Long 1979, ref. 105). Such inter-authority comparisons can have an odious aspect, and although not explicitly political, they may have political repercussions for some of the authorities compared (Eddison 1979, ref. 85). Identification of high and low-spending authorities may provoke demands for reduction in levels of spending and service provision to a mean, if not to the lowest common denominator.

Conversely, interest groups pursuing the entitlement of particular client groups to services may expose authorities whom they consider to be unsympathetic or out of line in order, presumably, to shame them into changing their attitude. In this case, a comparative approach is used to demonstrate geographical variations in policy and services, usually as between local authorities, but rarely to explain such variations. Some of this literature is based on academic research, but mostly it comes from pressure groups whose purpose is to campaign for change in legislation or in its implementation by local authorities. Thus Shelter has published numerous studies comparing local authority homelessness services, not always based on systematic surveys. These pressure groups would no doubt recognise a common purpose in their researches, although they appear not to be aware of each other's work, being interested in different client groups or policy areas.

The final category of literature is the most amorphous. It includes numerous unconnected studies of aspects of the health and personal social services (there must be many more than are listed here). In these, different geographical areas are likely to be studied within a conventional social science research framework, constituting, for example, a control group, or parts of a quota or stratified sample constructed on a geographical basis (Packman 1968, ref. 149). Sometimes these studies are less obviously systematic, and the selection of areas may appear to be haphazard. Many of these authors probably would not regard a comparative perspective as being central to their work, and they are the least likely among the groups I have outlined, to see themselves as contributing to a comparative discipline.

In constructing this bibliography, a decision had to be made on the selection of 'areas' which were being compared. Dimensions of comparison include: north–south; urban–rural; inner city and outer; adjacent or distant neighbourhoods; areas defined in positive discrimination programmes; administrative areas of local and regional government, most obviously local authorities at county or district level, and area health authorities. I have drawn the line at comparisons between institutions, such as hospitals. Although these are physically separate, the locational element seems secondary to organisational dimensions. It is, of course, possible to orientate comparative research around almost any two or more variables featuring in a cross-tabulation. These other ways of differentiating data and phenomena, for example by social class, gender, race, housing tenure, income or client group, may have geographical aspects, but unless these are primary and explicit, such studies have been excluded from the present bibliography.

Organisation

The titles listed in this bibliography (317 references) were published mainly during the 1970s, and up to February 1982. While mainly British, a few American references have been included – to literature involving comparisons between areas within the United States. These should add a useful dimension to the study of British domestic comparative social administration. No claims are made to comprehensiveness, and the bibliography should rather be regarded as a preliminary exercise.

The bibliography is organised in three sections. The first lists literature with an explicit comparative orientation, subdivided into general categories. These include appropriate theoretical frameworks and methods of analysis, not all of which are specifically applied to the health and personal social services.

Section two includes references to systematically presented data on the health and personal social services, where the focus is comparison between, or classification of, individual authorities. The standard data issued annually by the DHSS in *Health and Personal Social Services Statistics* and in *Social Trends* are not thus broken down. It should be noted that some of the sources listed may be cut under the Thatcher government's programme of reduction in central statistical services.

The third, and largest, section includes literature that is specific to client groups or services and whose authors may or may not regard the comparative dimension as the main focus of their work, as discussed above. There is necessarily some limited repetition of titles listed in section one. The classification followed within section three, and the style of referencing throughout, is adopted from my *Personal social services bibliography*, published by the Library Association to whom acknowledgement is therefore due.[5]

Notes

1. J. Baker, 'Social conscience and social policy', *Journal of Social Policy*, Vol. 8, no. 2, pp. 177–206.
2. J. Higgins, *States of welfare: comparative analysis in social policy*, Oxford: Blackwell, 1981; B. Q. Madison, *The meaning of social policy: the comparative dimensions in social welfare*, London: Croom Helm, 1980.
3. D. Donnison, *Social policy and administration revisited*, London: Allen and Unwin, 1975; P. Taylor-Gooby, 'The empiricist tradition in social administration, *Critical social policy*, Vol. 1, no. 2, pp. 6–21.
4. Department of Health and Social Security, *Priorities for health and personal social services in England*, London: HMSO, 1976, pp. 8–9.
5. G. Stewart, *Personal social services bibliography*, London: Library Association, 1980.

Bibliography Contents

Bibliography

Section one Explicitly comparative

I Theoretical frameworks, methods of analysis, studies with general application

1 Alt, J. E. 1977, 'Politics and expenditure models', *Policy and Politics*, Vol. 5, no. 3, pp. 83–92: influence of local political activity on local authority policy and expenditure on the social services.

2. Bennett, R. J. 1980, *The geography of public finance: welfare under fiscal federalism and local government finance*, Methuen.

3 Boal, F. W. and Douglas, J. N. H. 1982, *Integration and division: geographical perspectives on the Northern Ireland problem*, Academic Press: 'establishes cultural integration and division in plural societies as a general framework'.

4 Cox, K. R. 1973, *Conflict, power and politics in the city: a geographical view*, McGraw Hill.

5 Davidson, R. N. 1981, *Crime and environment*, Croom Helm: geographical and environmental distribution of incidence of reported crime.

6 Dicken, P. and Lloyd, P. E. 1981. *Modern western society: a geographical perspective on work, home and well-being*, Harper and Row.

7 Donnison, D. and Soto, P. 1980, 'Social policy goes spatial', in D. Donnison and P. Soto, *The good city: a study of urban development and policy in Britain*, Heinemann, Chapter 3, pp. 27–37.

8 Haggett, P. 1965, *Locational analysis in human geography*, Edward Arnold: discusses methodological problems in selection of areas to be compared.

9 Harvey, D. 1973, *Social justice and the city*, Edward Arnold, Chapters 1 and 2 'Social processes and spatial form'.

10 Herbert, D. 1982, *The geography of urban crime*, Longman: 'examines the data bases for the study of crime, the theories of criminology, the areal and ecological dimensions of criminality, the patterns of offences and problem areas, and concludes with an assessment of the directions of research and policy implications'; examples from South Wales.

11 Herbert, D. T. and Smith, D. M. (eds.) 1979, *Social problems and the city: geographical perspectives*, Oxford University Press.

12 Johnston, R. J. 1979, *Political, electoral and spatial systems*, Oxford University Press: 'presents a systematic view of the interrelationships between geographical and political variables and emphasises their consequences for the geography of inequality and the nature of democracy. Main argument is that geographical variation in the level of economic and social well-being results

from the electoral activities of political parties competing to gain and retain power. The main aspects of electoral geography dealt with are: the relationships between government and social well-being; the main elements of the electoral system; the geography of spending; local government reform; and the reorganisation and manipulation of electoral systems.' By the Professor of Geography, University of Sheffield.

13 Kamenka, E. (ed.) 1981, *Community*, Edward Arnold.

14 Knox, P. 1981, *Urban social geography: an introduction*, Longman.

15 Knox, P. L. and Cottam, M. B. 1981, 'A welfare approach to rural geography: contrasting perspectives on the quality of highland life', *Transactions Institute of British Geographers*, new series, Vol. 6, no. 4, pp. 433–50: compares Ullapool and Evanton.

16 Leach, B. 1980, *The social geography of urban youth*, Edward Arnold.

17 Le Grand, J. and Winter, D. 1977, 'Towards an economic model of local government behaviour', *Policy and Politics*, Vol. 5 no. 3, pp. 23–39.

18 Lewis, P. *et al.* (eds.) 1978, *The practice of comparative politics*, Longman, 2nd edn.: general political science perspectives; Open University set book.

19 Moore, N. and Leach, S. 1979, 'An interaction approach to county/district relationships', *Policy and Politics*, Vol. 7, no. 3, pp. 271–97.

20 Muir, R. and Paddison, R. 1981, *Politics, geography and behaviour*, Methuen.

21 Newton, K. and Sharpe, L. J. 1977, 'Local outputs research: some reflections and proposals', *Policy and Politics*, Vol. 5, no. 3, pp. 61–82: influence of non-political characteristics on policy variations at local government level.

22 Osborn, A. F. and Carpenter, A. P. 1980, 'A rating of neighbourhood types', *Clearing House for Local Authority Social Services Research*, no. 3, pp. 1–37: classification of four types of neighbourhood.

23 Rural Geography Study Group 1981, *Social problems in rural communities*, Institute of British Geographers: seminar papers.

24 Smith, C. J. 1980, 'social networks as metaphors, models and methods', *Progress in Human Geography*, Vol. 4, no. 4, pp. 500–24.

25 Warnes, A. M. (ed.) 1982, *Geographical perspectives on the elderly*, John Wiley.

26 Warnes, A. M. 1981, 'Towards a geographical contribution to gerontology', *Progress in Human Geography*, Vol. 5, no. 3, pp. 317–41.

27 Warren, D. I. 1978, 'Explorations in neighbourhood differentiation', *Sociological Quarterly*, Vol. 19, pp. 310–331.

28 Warren, D. I. 1981, *Helping networks: how people cope with problems in an urban community*, Dunlop: identifies types of neighbourhood, in USA.

29 Webster, B. and Stewart, J. 1974, 'The area analysis of resources', *Policy and Politics*, Vol. 3, no. 1, pp. 5–16: reviews literature and discusses research problems.

30 Weinstein, M. S. 1980, *Health in the city: environmental and behavioural influences*, Pergamon: American.

II Urban analysis, area programmes, 'need' and deprivation indicators

31 Bebbington, A. C. and Davies, B. 1980, 'Territorial need indicators: a new approach', *Journal of Social Policy*, Vol. 9, no. 2, pp. 145–68 and Vol. 9, no. 4, pp. 433–62.

32 Berthoud, R. *et al.* 1981, *Poverty and the development of anti-poverty policy in the UK*, Heinemann: ineffectiveness of area-based positive discrimination; part of the EEC anti-poverty programme.

33 Berthoud, R. 1982, 'United Kingdom?', *New Society*, 14 January 1982, pp. 56–57: poverty in Northern Ireland, compared with England.

34 Berthoud, R. 1976, 'Where are London's poor?', *Greater London Intelligence Journal*, no. 36, pp. 5–12: argues against the notion of deprivation being concentrated in geographical areas; evidence that low income is not clustered at ward level.

35 Blowers, A. *et al*. 1982, *Urban change and conflict: an interdisciplinary reader*, Harper and Row.

36 Boaden, N. 1971, *Urban policy-making*, Cambridge University Press: political science perspective on variations in expenditure between different local authorities.

37 Boviard, A. G. (ed.) 1978, *Research and intelligence for deprivation*, University of Birmingham: Liverpool, Nottinghamshire and Strathclyde; the area approach to deprivation and positive discrimination.

38 Butler, P. and Williams, R. H. 1981, 'Inner city partnerships and established policies', *Policy and Politics*, Vol. 9, no. 2, pp. 125–36.

39 Cameron, G. (ed.) 1980, *The future of the British conurbations: policies and prescriptions for change*, Longman.

40 Carley, M. 1981, *Social measurement and social indicators*, George Allen and Unwin.

41 Cleworth, P. 1977, 'Positive discrimination and urban deprivation', *Local Government Studies*, Vol. 3, no. 3, pp. 23–25.

42 Cox, K. R. 1973, *Conflict, power and politics in the city: a geographic view*, McGraw Hill.

43 Davies, B. 1977, 'Social service studies and the explanation of policy outcomes', *Policy and Politics*, Vol. 5, no. 3, pp. 41–59: relevant to 'need' indicators.

44 Department of the Environment 1977, *Inner area studies: Liverpool, Birmingham and Lambeth – summaries of consultants' final reports*, HMSO.

45 Donnison, D. 1974, 'Policies for priority areas', *Journal of Social Policy*, Vol. 3, no. 2.

46 Edwards, J. 1973, 'Social indicators, urban deprivation and positive discrimination', *Journal of Social Policy*, Vol. 2, no. 3.

47 Edwards, J. 1975, *Urban deprivation and stress indices*, Centre for Urban and Regional Studies, University of Birmingham.

48 Flynn, M. *et al*. 1973, 'Social malaise research: a study in Liverpool', *Social Trends*, Vol. 4, pp. 42–52: locating areas of deprivation within the city.

49 Goldsmith, M. 1981, *Politics, planning and the city*, Hutchinson: examples from social services, planning and housing.

50 Gordon, I. 1977, 'Subjective social indicators and urban political analysis: or, what do we need to know about who's happy?', *Policy and Politics*, Vol. 5, no. 3, pp. 93–111.

51 Hall, P. (ed.) 1981, *The inner city in context: the final report of the SSRC inner cities working party*, Heinemann.

52 Hall, P. 1980, 'Two nations or one: the geography of deprivation', *New Society*, 14 February 1980: north/south inequality.

53 Hambleton, R. 1977, 'Policies for areas', *Local Government Studies*, Vol. 3, no. 2, pp. 13–29.

54 Hatch, S. and Sherrott, R. 1973, 'Positive discrimination and the distribution of deprivations', *Policy and Politics*, Vol. 1, no. 3, pp. 223–40.

55 Herbert, D. T. and Johnson, R. J. (eds.) 1981. *Geography and the urban environment: progress in research and applications*, John Wiley.

56 Herbert, D. T. and Smith, D. M. (eds.) 1979, *Social problems and the city*, Oxford University Press: Chapter 2 on social indicators; Chapters 12 and 13 on area-based policies for inner cities.

57 Holterman, S. 1975, 'Areas of urban deprivation in Great Britain', *Social Trends*, Vol. 6.

58 Holterman, S. 1975, *Census indicators of urban deprivation*, Department of the Environment.

59 Imber, V. 1977, 'Expenditure on the personal social services and area classification of need', *Social Services Research Group Journal*, no. 1: by OPCS researcher, see ref. 128.

60 Jenkins, J. and Rose, M. 1976, 'Rate support grants and their application to London', *Greater London Intelligence Quarterly*, no. 35, pp. 9–25: includes calculation of the needs element.

61 Knox, P. and Cottam, B. 1981, 'Rural deprivation in Scotland: a preliminary assessment', *Tijdschrift voor Economische en Sociale Geografie*, Vol. 72, no. 3, pp. 162–75: areal analysis of deprivation indicators.

62 Maclaran, A. 1981, 'Area-based positive discrimination and the distribution of well-being', *Transactions Institute of British Geographers* new series, Vol. 6, no. 1, pp. 53–67: areal analysis in Dundee.

63 Mason, T. *et al.* 1977, *Tackling urban deprivation: the contribution of area-based management*, INLOGOV, University of Birmingham.

64 Northern Ireland Office 1976, *Belfast: areas of special social need. Report by project team*, HMSO.

65 Orr, L. C. 1975, *Income, employment and urban residential location*, Academic Press.

66 Robson, B. T. 1969, *Urban analysis: a study of city structure*, Cambridge University Press.

67 Shonfield, A. and Shaw, S. (eds.) 1972, *Social indicators and social policy*, Heinemann.

68 Smith, D. L. 1978, 'Policy-making for urban deprivation', *Public Administration*, Vol. 56, pp. 193–202: DoE author considers justification for coordinated area approach; discusses difficulties, particularly in identification, and choice of style and scale.

69 Townsend, P. 1976, 'Area deprivation policies', *New Statesman*, 6 August 1976, pp. 168–71.

70 Townsend, P. 1979, *Poverty in the United Kingdom*, Penguin Books; Chapter 15, 'The problems of poor areas', pp. 543–64.

71 Turner, J. 1977, 'Salubrious Solihull', *New Society*, 10 November 1977, pp. 301–2: the good life in Solihull compared with deprivation indicators for Islington.

72 Vielba, C. A. 1978, 'Does the area approach work?', *Municipal Review*, Vol. 48, no. 578, pp. 344–45: institutional hindrances to positive discrimination programmes in inner cities.

73 *Political Quarterly* 1981, Vol. 52, no. 1: whole issue on unemployment, mostly from regional perspectives.

III Resource allocation, territorial (in)justice, inter-authority comparison

74 Association of Directors of Social Services 1980, *Cuts in public expenditure: the effects on the personal social services*, Newcastle-upon-Tyne, ADSS.

75 Bebbington, A. and Davies, B. 1977, 'What difference have the cuts made?', *Social Work Today*, 27 September 1977, pp. 6–7.

76 Brown, M. 1981, *Personal social services expenditure in staffing and activities*, Newcastle-upon-Tyne, ADSS: survey of eighty-two local social services authorities in England and Wales analyses effects of cuts in public expenditure.

77 Buxton, M. J. and Klein, R. E. 1978, *Allocating health resources: a commentary on the report of the Resource Allocation Working Party*, HMSO, Royal Commission on the National Health Service Research Paper no. 3.

78 Coutts, I. 1979, 'Cuts and costs', *County Councils Gazette*, Vol. 72, no. 6, pp. 180–81: regional differences in service provision; aim for the lowest common denominator.

79 Davies B. 1968, *Social needs and resources in local services*, Michael Joseph: first statement of Davies' theories on territorial injustice.

80 Davies, B. 1977, 'Social service studies and the explanation of policy outcomes', *Policy and Politics*, Vol. 5, no. 3, pp. 41–59: relevant to territorial justice.

81 Davies, B. 1976, 'Territorial injustice', *New Society*, 13 May 1976.

82 Davies, B. *et al.* 1972, *Variations in children's services among British urban authorities*, Bell.

83 Davies, B. *et al.* 1971, 'Variations in the provision of local authority health and welfare services for the elderly: a comparison between counties and county boroughs', *Social and Economic Administration*, Vol. 5, no. 2, pp. 100–24.

84 Davies, B. *et al.* 1971, *Variations in services for the aged*, Bell: between local authorities.

85 Eddison, T. 1979, 'Inter-authority comparisons – an irrelevant extravaganza?', *Municipal Journal*, 14 December 1979, pp. 1314–5: SAUS director attacks the fashion for comparing local authorities' performance and expenditure, part 1.

86 Eddison, T. 1979, 'An alternative approach to inter-authority comparisons', *Municipal Journal*, 21 December 1979, pp. 1346–7: part 2 of the article.

87 Falk, N. and Webb, A. 1975, 'After the plans', *New Society*, 11 September 1975, pp. 585–6: how ten social services departments went about creating their ten-year plans.

88 Foster, C. and Lynch, B. 1977, 'Local cuts are private', *New Society*, 10 March 1977, p. 500: effects on local government of public expenditure cuts; by the director of CES.

89 Hambleton, R. 1977, 'A guideline is a trap', *New Society*, 24 March 1977, p. 601: local authorities' attitudes to central government guidelines.

90 Hambleton, R. 1978, *Policy planning and local government*, Hutchinson: includes local studies of Liverpool and Stockport.

91 Hambleton, R. and Scerri, V. 1974, 'Three social services plans compared', *Clearing House for Local Authority Social Services Research*, no. 1, pp. 61–8: Salford, Hackney and Cheshire.

92 Hambleton, R. and Scerri, V. 1973, 'Three views of need', *New Society*, 18 October 1973, pp. 146–7: compares social services ten year plans for Salford, Hackney and Cheshire.

93 Harvey, D. 1973, *Social justice and the city*, Edward Arnold: chapter 3, 'Social justice and spatial systems', including 'Terrirorial distributive justice'.

94 Herbert, D. T. and Smith, D. M. (eds.) 1979, *Social problems and the city*, Oxford University Press: Chapters 1, 3 and 4 on resource allocation.

95 Imber, V. 1977, 'Expenditure on the personal social services and area classification of need', *Social Services Research Group Journal*, no. 1, October 1977: by OPCS researcher, see ref. 128.
96 Jackman, R. 1978, 'Assessing rates needs', *New Society*, 12 January 1978, p. 72: needs element in the rate support grant to city authorities.
97 Jackson, M. P. *et al*. 1979, 'Variations in the provision of financial aid through social work in Scottish local authorities', *Policy and Politics*, Vol. 7, no. 1, pp. 69–81.
98 Jenkins, R. and Rose, M. 1976, 'Rate support grants and their application to London', *Greater London Intelligence Quarterly*, no. 35, pp. 9–25: includes calculation of the needs element.
99 Jones, D. and Bourne, A. 1976, 'Monitoring the distribution of resources in the NHS', *Social and Economic Administration*, Vol. 10, no. 2, pp. 92–105.
100 Judge, K. 1978, *Rationing social services*, Heinemann: general book with relevant sections, including one on territorial injustice.
101 Judge, K. 1974, 'The social services: where the money goes', *New Society*, 8 August 1974, p. 343: effect of public expenditure cuts on personal social services budgets in seven counties.
102 Judge, K. 1975, 'Territorial justice and local authority loan sanctions in the personal social services', *Policy and Politics*, Vol. 3, no. 4, pp. 43–70.
103 Kahan, B. 1968, 'Children "in care"', *New Society*, 2 May 1968, p. 643: territorial injustice in children's services.
104 Knapp, P. 1980, 'Penny a minute', *Community Care*, 20 March 1980, pp. 18–19: national survey of observation and assessment centres for children in local authority care; particularly differential expenditure between local authorities.
105 Long, J. (ed.) 1979, *Inter-authority comparisons: a report by the Institute of Local Government Studies on a seminar sponsored by SOLACE*, CURS, University of Birmingham.
106 Maynard, A. and Ludbrook, A. 1980, 'Budget allocation in the National Health Service', *Journal of Social Policy*, Vol. 9, no. 3, pp. 289–312: resource allocation and geographical inequality.
107 Meacher, M. 1971, 'Scrooge areas', *New Society*, 2 December 1971.
108 Minors, M. and Kenny, D. 1976, *Personal social services: estimated net revenue expenditure on client groups*, Greater London Council Research Memo no. 484: among the London boroughs.
109 Moseley, L. G. 1968, 'Variations in socio-medical services for the aged', *Social and Economic Administration*, Vol. 2, no. 3.
110 Nicholson, R. J. and Topham, N. 1972, 'Investment decisions and the size of local authorities', *Policy and Politics*, Vol. 1, no. 1, pp. 23–44.
111 Pinch, S. 1979, 'Territorial justice in the city: a case study of the social services for the elderly in Greater London', in D. T. Herbert and D. M. Smith (eds.) 1979, *Social problems and the city*, Oxford University Press, Chapter 11, pp. 201–223.
112 Resource Allocation Working Party (DHSS) 1976, *Sharing resources for health in England*, HMSO: regional variations in health service resources.
113 Wandsworth Social Services Department 1978, 'Area spending', *Clearing House for Local Authority Social Services Research*, no. 4, pp. 55–72: 'a geographical look at spending in six social work areas, highlighting differences between each without necessarily trying to explain them'.

114 Wandsworth Social Services Department 1977, 'Cutting the joint finance cake', *Clearing House for Local Authority Social Services Research*, no. 5, pp. 1–28: nine different methods of an Area Health Authority allocating joint funding money between three local authorities in south London.

115 Wandsworth Social Services Department 1976, 'Wandsworth comparatively speaking', *Clearing House for Local Authority Social Services Research*, no. 4, pp. 1–80: inner London boroughs' provision of personal social services compared, using DHSS statistics.

116 Wandsworth Social Services Department 1976, *Wandsworth . . . comparatively speaking again*, London Borough of Wandsworth: comparing personal social services in Wandsworth with other inner London boroughs, repeat exercise.

117 Webb, A. and Falk, N. 1974, 'Planning the social services: the local authority ten year plans', *Policy and Politics*, Vol. 3, no. 2, pp. 33–54: uses ten published plans and a small survey of London social services departments.

118 Weir, S. and Simpson, R. 1980, 'Are the local authority social services being bled dry?', *New Society*, 10 July 1980, pp. 59–62: survey of implementation of cuts in all social services departments in England and Wales, April 1980.

119 1973, 'Assessing the cuts', *New Society*, 25 October 1973, p. 215: estimating effects of public expenditure cuts on local services generally.

Section two

IV Statistical sources

120 Chartered Institute of Public Finance and Accountancy 1981, *Local Government comparative statistics 1981*, CIPFA: actuals and estimates, authorities identified; introduction discusses compilation and use of comparative statistics.

121 Chartered Institute of Public Finance and Accountancy 1981, *Personal social services statistics 1979–81 actuals*, CIPFA: and annually since 1976; local authorities' spending, based on voluntary returns so not comprehensive.

122 Department of Health and Social Security, *Health and personal social services statistics for England*, HMSO: annually since 1972 one year in arrears; identifies Regional Health Authorities only in few tables.

123 Department of Health and Social Security, *Health and personal social services statistics for Wales*, HMSO: annually since 1974 one year in arrears; identifies Area Health Authorities only in few tables.

124 Department of Health and Social Security *et al.*, *Hospital in-patient enquiry*, HMSO: annually, published three–four years in arrears; three vols. 'Maternity tables', 'Preliminary tables', 'Main tables'; based on one in ten sample of hospital in-patients; identifies regions, England and Wales.

125 Hale, R. 1977, 'Our needy urban areas', *New Society*, 18 August 1977, p. 346: about the DHSS's classification of the English social services authorities.

126 Howe, G. M. (Royal Geographical Society) 1970, *National atlas of disease mortality in the United Kingdom*, Nelson, revised edition: identifies regions and towns, includes maps.

127 Hutton, D. S. S. *et al.* 1974, 'Personal social services statistics', *Journal of the Royal Statistical Society*, series A, Vol. 137, no. 4: using the local authorities' returns.

128 Imber, V. 1977, *A classification of the English personal social services authorities*, HMSO, DHSS Statistical and Research Report Series no. 16.

129 Office of Population Censuses and Surveys 1974, *Morbidity statistics from general practice: second national study 1970–71*, HMSO: identifies standard regions.
130 Office of Population Censuses and Surveys 1980, *People in Britain: a census atlas*, HMSO: visual aspects of demography.
131 Webber, R. and Craig, J. 1978, *Socio-economic classification of local authority areas*, HMSO, OPCS Studies on Medical and Population Subjects no. 35.
132 1968, *Report of the committee on local authority and allied personal social services* (Seebohm report), Cmnd 3703, HMSO: Appendix G, 'Unevenness of the extent of the provision in the health and welfare services among local authorities', pp. 310–317; Appendix H, 'Health and welfare services, committee and administrative arrangements in local authorities', pp. 318–21.

Section three Client group and service studies with a comparative dimension

V Children, young people and families
(refer to XIII Offenders, for literature on juvenile offenders)

133 Armistead, N. *et al*. 1975, *Children's day care facilities in London 1966–74*, Greater London Council Research Memo. no. 472.
134 Armstrong, G. *et al*. 1980, *Mentally handicapped under-fives: Leeds and Sheffield services as seen by parents*, Evaluation Research Group Report no. 8, University of Sheffield.
135 Bacon, R. and Rowe, J. 1978, *Substitute family care – a regional study: the use and misuse of resources*, Association of British Adoption and Fostering Agencies.
136 Blackstone, T. 1969, 'Where nursery schools are', *New Society*, 9 October 1969, pp. 560–61: compares local authorities' provision.
137 Bone, M. 1978, *The family planning services: changes and effects*, HMSO: OPCS survey.
138 Bone, M. 1977, *Pre-school children and the need for day care*, HMSO: OPCS survey.
139 Child Guidance Special Interest Group 1975, *The child guidance service: a survey 1969*, Birmingham, British Association of Social Workers.
140 Davies, B. *et al*. 1972, *Variations in children's services among British urban authorities*, Bell.
141 Davies, H. and Plank, D. 1975, *Children in the care of the London boroughs 1967–1973*, Greater London Council Research Memo. no. 480.
142 House of Commons Social Services Committee 1980, *Perinatal and neonatal mortality*, HC 663–1, HMSO: regional variations.
143 Kahan, B. 1968, 'Children "in care"', *New Society*, 2 May 1968, p. 643: territorial injustice in children's services.
144 Knapp, M. 1980, 'Penny a minute', *Community Care*, 20 March 1980, pp. 18–19: national survey of observation and assessment centres for children in local authority care; particularly differential expenditure between local authorities.
145 Knox, E. G. *et al*. 1980, 'Social and health care determinants of area variations in perinatal mortality', *Community Medicine*, Vol. 2, no. 4, pp. 282–90.
146 Leach, B. 1980, *The social geography of urban youth*, Edward Arnold.

147 London Council of Social Service 1977, *Childminding in London: a study of support services for childminders*, LCSS: London boroughs.

148 Moss, P. *et al.* 1973, 'Families and their needs', *New Society*, 22 March 1973, p. 638: use of health and personal social services by mothers of pre-school children in Kirby and a London borough.

149 Packman, J. 1968, *Child care: needs and numbers*, George Allen and Unwin: study of practice in fifty local authorities, 'selected on the basis of a stratified sample which took account of geographical location, county or county borough status and numbers in care.' Authorities are named.

150 Rogers, S. and Titterington, J. 1978, *A survey of non-accidental injury registers in Northern Ireland*, Ulster Polytechnic.

151 Seed, P. and Thomson, M. 1978, *All kinds of care: an investigation into the use of residential and day care facilities for children in the highlands and western islands of Scotland*, Department of Social Work, University of Aberdeen, 2nd edition.

152 Shinman, S. M. 1981, *A chance for every child? Access and response to pre-school provision*, Tavistock.

VI Day and domiciliary services

153 Bolton, G. 1980, 'Prevention: an exploratory study of health visiting in England, Wales and Scotland', *Health Visitor*, Vol. 53, no. 6, pp. 203–6.

154 Carter, J. 1981, *Day services for adults*, George Allen and Unwin: five-year national survey; three volumes of data available from NISW.

155 Davies, B. and Coles O. 1981, 'Towards a territorial cost function for the home help service', *Social Policy and Administration*, Vol. 15, no. 1, pp. 32–42.

156 Hunt, A. 1970, *The home help service in England and Wales*, HMSO: OPCS survey.

157 Kenny, D. 1977, *Home help service in London 1966–75*, Greater London Council Research Memo. no. 518: London boroughs.

158 Means, R. 1981, *'Community care' and meals on wheels: a study in the politics of service development at the national and local level*, SAUS, University of Bristol.

159 National Council of Home Help Services n.d. (1978), *Home help services in Great Britain*, National Council of Home Help Services: extensive tables.

160 PA Management Consultants 1974, *Meals on wheels: short-term study*, a report to DHSS by PA Management Consultants Ltd.

161 Randall, G. W. *et al.* 1973, 'Area distribution of resources in Coventry', *Local Government Finance*, no. 11, pp. 396–400: relevant to home helps, branch libraries and maternal and child health clinics.

162 Speak, M. and Aitken-Swan, J. 1982, *Male midwives: a report on two studies*, DHSS: in Forth Valley, Scotland and London Borough of Islington.

163 Stapenhurst, P. 1978. *The home help service, the meals service in greater London*, Greater London Association for the Disabled.

VII Disabled people

164 Bowl, R. 1976, 'A survey of surveys', *New Society*, 28 October 1976, p. 195: Chronically Sick and Disabled Persons Act 1970, need identification surveys, as conducted in different local authority areas.

165 Brown, M. J. and Bowl, R. 1976, *Study of local authority chronic sick and disabled persons surveys*, Birmingham, Social Services Research Group: with three volumes of appendices.

166 Browning, J. and Hope-Murray, E. L. 1974, 'Notes of developing local authority social services in England under the Chronically Sick and Disabled Persons Act', *Social Work Service*, no. 5, pp. 5–10.
167 Gregory, E. 1973, 'Implementing the Chronically Sick and Disabled Persons Act: review article', *Social Work Today*, 23 August 1973.
168 Harris, A. I. *et al.* 1971, *Handicapped and impaired in Great Britain*, Vol. 1, HMSO: OPCS survey, includes some comparison of services among authorities and regions.
169 Knight, R. and Warren, M. D. 1978, *Physically disabled people living at home: a study of numbers and needs*, HMSO, DHSS Report on Health and Social Services no. 13: 'based mainly on a study of the methods and results of surveys undertaken by social services departments of local authorities in accordance with the provisions of the Chronically Sick and Disabled Persons Act 1970; from the Health Services Research Unit at University of Kent.
170 Lowther, C. P. *et al.* 1973, *Studies in disability in Exeter and Edinburgh*, University of Exeter.
171 Mole, S. 1979, 'The good, the bad and the ignorant', *Community Care*, 18 January 1979, pp. 28–30: vagueness in the Chronically Sick and Disabled Persons Act 1970 encourages a low and uneven level of implementation by local authorities; tables of named authorities.
172 Sainsbury, S. 1970, *Registered as disabled*, Bell, Occasional Papers on Social Administration no. 35: interviews with 211 registered disabled people in London, Essex and Middlesex, on their living conditions and services received. Appendix 3 tabulates 'Variations between local authorities in their provision for physically handicapped persons'.
173 Scottish Council on Disability 1978, *Accommodation for the disabled in Scotland: a survey of provision, needs and resources*, Edinburgh, Scottish Council on Disability.
174 Social Policy Research 1973, *The implementation of the Chronically Sick and Disabled Persons Act*, National Fund for Research Into Crippling Diseases.

VIII Elderly people

175 Age Concern Research Unit 1981, *Profiles of the elderly 6.8, their use of the social services*, Age Concern: local variations.
176 Bowl, R. *et al* 1979, 'Not just a day out', *Community Care*, 14 June 1979, pp. 26–27: day care for the elderly in Kirklees, Birmingham and East Anglia, from DHSS funded research.
177 Brocklehurst, J. C. 1970, *The geriatric day hospital: a report of three studies of geriatric day hospitals in Great Britain and Northern Ireland*, King's Fund Centre.
178 Davies, B. *et al.* 1971, 'Variations in the provision of local authority health and welfare services for the elderly: a comparison between counties and county boroughs', *Social and Economic Administration*, Vol. 5, no. 2, pp. 100–124.
179 Davies, B. *et al.* 1971, *Variations in services for the aged*, Bell: between local authorities.
180 Department of Health and Social Security, Social Work Service, London Region 1979, *Residential care for the elderly in London*, DHSS SWS.
181 Flynn, M. L. 1980, 'Coordination of social and health care for the elderly: the British and Irish examples', *The Gerontologist*, Vol. 20, no. 3, part I, pp. 300–07.

182 Hall, A. and Wicks, M. 1975, 'Winning the cold war for old people', *Community Care*, 11 June 1975, pp. 14–18: survey of London boroughs' provision for cold old people.

183 Harris, A. 1968, *Social welfare for the elderly: a study in thirteen local authority areas in England, Wales and Scotland*, HMSO, 2 vols.: OPCS survey.

184 Hunt, A. 1978, *The elderly at home: a study of people aged sixty five and over living in the community in England in 1976*, HMSO: OPCS survey, includes some comparison between regions.

185 Karn, V. A. 1977, *Retiring to the seaside*, Routledge & Kegan Paul: compares the situation of and provision for old people in Bexhill-on-Sea and Clacton.

186 Moseley, L. G. 1968, 'Variations in socio-medical services for the aged', *Social and Economic Administration*, Vol. 2, no. 3.

187 Nelson, G. 1980, 'Social services to the urban and rural aged: the experience of area agencies on ageing', *The Gerontologist*, Vol. 20, no. 2, pp. 200–07: level of service is lower in rural areas; American.

188 Newman, R. and Bacon, V. 1980, *Report on a survey of housing for old people provided by local authorities and housing associations in England and Wales*, Department of the Environment.

189 Pinch, S. 1979, 'Territorial justice in the city: a case study of the social services for the elderly in Greater London', in D. T. Herbert and D. M. Smith (eds.) 1979, *Social problems and the city*, Oxford University Press: Chapter 11, pp. 201–23.

190 Plank, D. 1977, *Caring for the elderly: report on a study of various means of caring for dependent elderly people in eight London boroughs*, Greater London Council Research Memo. no. 512.

191 Snow, T. 1981, *Services for old age*, Age Concern: compares levels of health and personal social services provision in London with the rest of England.

192 Stanton, B. R. 1971, *Meals for the elderly: a report on meals on wheels and luncheon clubs in two north London boroughs*, King's Fund Centre.

193 Sumner, G. and Smith, R. 1969, *Planning local authority services for the elderly*, George Allen and Unwin: in forty-one local authority areas.

194 Townsend, P. 1964, *The last refuge: a survey of residential institutions and homes for the aged in England and Wales*, Routledge and Kegan Paul.

195 Townsend, P. 1963, 'The timid and the bold', *New Society*, 23 May 1963, pp. 16–18: local authority plans for services for the elderly, in connection with Cmnd 1973; tables of named authorities.

196 Wan, T. T. H. and Odell, B. G. 1981, 'Factors affecting the use of social and health services among the elderly', *Ageing and Society*, Vol. 1, no. 1, pp. 95–115: geographical location is one factor.

197 Warnes, A. M. (ed.) 1982, *Geographical perspectives on the elderly*, John Wiley.

198 Warnes, A. M. 1981, 'Towards a geographical contribution to gerontology', *Progress in Human Geography*, Vol. 5 no. 3, pp. 317–41.

IX Health services

199 Bolden, K. 1981, *Inner cities*, Royal College of General Practitioners, Occasional Paper 19: survey of GPs in nine cities.

200 Bolton, G. 1980, 'Prevention: an exploratory study of health visiting in England, Wales and Scotland', *Health Visitor*, Vol. 53, no. 6, pp. 203–06.

201 Buxton, M. J. and Klein, R. E. 1978, *Allocating health resources: a commentary on the report of the Resource Allocation Working Party*, HMSO, Royal Commission on the National Health Service Research Paper no. 3.

202 Department of Health and Social Security (Black Committee) 1980, *Inequalities in health: report of a research working group*, DHSS.

203 Hassinger, E. W. *et al*. 1980, 'Perceptions of rural and metropolitan physicians about rural practice and the rural community, Missouri, 1975' *Public Health Reports*, Vol. 95, no. 1, pp. 69–79: American.

204 House of Commons Social Services Committee 1980, *Perinatal and neonatal mortality*, HC663–1, HMSO: regional variations.

205 Jones, D. and Bourne, A. 1976, 'Monitoring the distribution of resources in the NHS', *Social and Economic Administration*, Vol. 10, no. 2, pp. 92–105.

206 Knox, E. G. *et al*. 1980, 'Social and health care determinants of area variation in perinatal mortality', *Community Medicine*, Vol. 2, no. 4, pp. 282–90.

207 Maynard, A. and Ludbrook, A. 1980, 'Budget allocation in the National Health Service', *Journal of Social Policy*, Vol. 9, no. 3, pp. 289–312: resource allocation and geographical inequality.

208 Resource Allocation Working Party (DHSS) 1976, *Sharing resources for health in England*, HMSO: regional variations in health service resources.

209 Simpson, R. 1979, *Access to primary care*, HMSO, Royal Commission on the National Health Service Research Paper no. 6: consumer opinion about general practitioners in Stoke Newington (north London) and Cockermouth, by a National Consumer Council researcher.

210 Speak, M. and Aitken-Swan, J. 1982, *Male midwives: a report on two studies*, DHSS: in Forth Valley, Scotland and London Borough of Islington.

211 Townsend, P. 1974, 'Inequality and the health service', *The Lancet*, 15 June 1974, pp. 1180–90.

212 Weinstein, M. S. 1980, *Health in the city: environmental and behavioural influences*, Pergamon: American.

X Homeless people: families, individuals, battered women

213 After Six *et al*. (Joint Charities Group) 1978, *The implementation of the Housing (Homeless Persons) Act, 1977: an appraisal after four months*, Shelter Housing Aid Centre: comparisons between various local authorities; anecdotal rather than systematic.

214 Bailey, R. and Ruddock, J. 1972, *Grief report: a Shelter report on temporary accommodation*, Shelter: compares local authorities' practices.

215 Bamford, T. 1975, 'Homelessness', *Social Work Today*, 20 March 1975, pp. 782–3: practice in twenty local authorities since DoE circular 18/74 recommended transfer of responsibility from social services departments to housing departments.

216 Barr, N. A. and Carrier, J. W. 1978, 'Women's aid groups: the economic case for state assistance to battered wives', *Policy and Politics*, Vol. 6, no. 3, pp. 333–50: investigates the Chiswick and Camden refuges, and their relationships with their respective local authorities; John Carrier is a Camden councillor.

217 Bates, P. 1974, *Single and homeless in Scotland: some facts*, Edinburgh, Grassmarket Project.

218 Billcliffe, S. 1979, 'Homeless, unintentional, priority – but dumped in the interim', *Roof*, July 1979, pp. 118–21: local authorities' use of 'interim' accommodation for homeless families, by a Shelter campaigner.

219 Billcliffe, S. 1978, *Where homelessness means hopelessness: an appraisal of the first year of the Housing (Homeless Persons) Act*, Shelter: compares English regions.

220 Binney, V. *et al.* 1981, *Leaving violent men: a study of refuges and housing for battered women*, Women's Aid Federation: survey shows incidence of refuges nationally, and local authorities' practices in rehousing; DoE funded research.

221 Campaign for the Homeless and Rootless 1973, *37/72: 33 local authorities one year after*, CHAR: non-implementation of the DHSS circular 37/72 on 'Homeless single persons in need of care and support'.

222 Chartered Institute of Public Finance and Accountancy 1980, *Homelessness statistics, 1978–79 actuals*, CIPFA: expenditure by housing authorities in England and Wales; authorities are identified but returns were voluntary and are therefore incomplete.

223 Diamond, G. 1975. *Homeless pregnant women*, After Six Housing Advisory Service: tabulated comparison between London boroughs' treatment of homeless pregnant women, see also ref. 236.

224 Drake, M. and Biebuych, T. 1977, *Policy and provision for the single homeless*, Personal Social Services Council: compares the situation in selected London boroughs, shire and metropolitan counties in England.

225 Drake, M. *et al.* 1981, *Single and homeless*, HMSO: survey of single homeless people and services in Camden, Tower Hamlets, Haringey, Manchester, Stoke-on Trent, Bedford and Brighton, conducted from CES and funded by DoE; pp. 13–14, 'Homelessness in different types of areas'; appendix II, 'Selection of survey areas and rates of homelessness in different areas'; appendix III, 'Summary description of the survey areas'.

226 Glastonbury, B. 1971, *Homeless near a thousand homes*, George Allen and Unwin: homeless families in Gloucester, Somerset and Bristol, commissioned by DHSS along with Greve on London, see ref. 227.

227 Greve, J. *et al.* 1971, *Homelessness in London*, Scottish Academic Press: London boroughs' treatment of homeless families, commissioned by DHSS along with Glastonbury on the south west, see ref. 226.

228 Harvey, A. 1974, 'April and the homeless', *New Society*, 21 March 1974, p. 707: territorial injustice and general inadequacies of local authorities' provision for homeless families, in the context of local government reorganisation.

229 Harvey, A. 1969, 'Homeless? You can't come here', *New Society*, 27 February 1969, p. 323: patterns of local authority welfare departments' provision for homeless families.

230 Hiro, D. 1976, 'Homeless: duties must be enforced', *Roof*, January 1976, pp. 7–10: if they can get away with it, some local authorities will evade responsibility by inventing exclusion categories.

231 Ivatts, J. 1979, *Homelessness and legislation: a study of the effects of the Housing (Homeless Persons) Act, 1977*, Department of Government, Brunel University: from an MA thesis, based on a questionnaire to housing depatments.

232 Kenny, D. and Thompson, Q. 1978, *Refuges for battered women in London: provision and need*, Greater London Council Research Memo. no. 537.

233 Local Authorities Management Services and Computer Committee 1978, *Homelessness*, LAMSAC: survey of local authority homelessness policies, commissioned by the local authority associations.

234 McConnachie, I. 1978, 'The management aspect', *Local Government Chronicle*, 16 June 1978, pp. 639–40: on the LAMSAC report, see ref. 233.

235 Minns, R. 1972, 'Homeless families and some organisational determinants of deviancy', *Policy and Politics*, Vol. 1, no. 1, pp. 1–22: compares London boroughs' practices, following Greve's study, see ref. 227.

236 Morris, R. 1975, 'Homeless parents', *New Society*, 14 August 1975, pp. 372–3: After Six's survey of London boroughs' treatment of homeless pregnant women, see ref. 223.
237 National Assistance Board 1966, *Homeless single persons*, HMSO: survey of people living in lodging houses, hostels and reception centres in Britain; compares towns.
238 National Women's Aid Federation 1978, *'Half the sky' and still no roof: a report on the Housing (Homeless Persons) Act, 1977*, NWAF: local authorities' treatment of homeless battered women.
239 Phillips, M. 1976, 'Homeless by whim', *New Society*, 7 October 1976: inequality in local authorities' implementation of DoE circular 18/74, based on an unpublished DoE survey.
240 Pryce, M. 1977, 'Local authorities defend their record on hostels', *Social Work Today*, 1 February 1977, p. 3: responses to accusations in a Shelter pamphlet, see ref. 243.
241 Scottish Homeless Group 1978, *Housing (Homeless Persons) Act, 1977: a review of the first six months*, Edinburgh, Shelter: local authorities' implementation of the Act in Scotland.
242 Shelter 1976, *Blunt powers, sharp practices: a survey of local authority policies on homelessness*, Shelter.
243 Shelter 1977, *Hostel for a home*, Shelter: survey of local authority hostel accommodation for homeless families.
244 Shelter 1977, *Insult to injury: homelessness policy in south Wales*, Bristol, Shelter: compares local authorities' policies and practices in south Wales.
245 Shelter Housing Aid Centre 1976, *Violence in marriage*, SHAC: London local housing authorities' policies concerning homeless battered women with children.
246 Stewart, G. and Stewart, J. 1978, 'The Housing (Homeless Persons) Act, 1977: a reassessment of social need', in M. Brown and S. Baldwin (eds.) 1978, *The year book of social policy in Britain, 1977*, Routledge and Kegan Paul: Chapter 2 includes a section on territorial injustice between local authorities' homelessness services, pp. 35–8.
247 Stewart, J. M. 1975, *Of no fixed abode: vagrancy and the welfare state*, Manchester University Press: compares the incidence of former lodging house residents in local authority old people's homes in four Lancashire welfare authority areas in 1970; based on an MA thesis.
248 Tai Nos 1978, *I ended up on my own with a torch: the Housing (Homeless Persons) Act 1977 in south Wales*, Cardiff, Tai Nos: compares various local authorities' practices in south Wales.
249 Welsh Women's Aid 1980, *Which venue now: a survey of the use of the Magistrates Court Act in Wales*, Cardiff, WWA.
250 Widdowson, B. 1981, *Intentional homelessness*, Shelter: survey of local housing authorities' operation of the discretionary clause in the Housing (Homeless Persons) Act, 1977.
251 Wingfield Digby, P. 1976, *Hostels and lodgings for single people*, HMSO: follow-up of the NAB survey ref. 237, with similar terms of reference; conducted from OPCS.

XI Material aid

252 Emmett, T. and Hawker, M. 1975, 'Section one money – a supplement to supplementary benefits', *Social Work Today*, 3 April 1975, p. 27: survey on

local authorities' use of financial powers under section one of the Children and Young Persons Act, 1963.

253 Heywood, J. S. and Allen, B. K. 1971, *Financial help in social work: a study of preventive work with families under the Children and Young Persons Act, 1963*, Manchester University Press: compares local authorities.

254 Hill, M. and Laing, P. 1978, *Money payments, social work and supplementary benefits: a study of section one of the 1963 Children and Young Persons Act*, SAUS, University of Bristol.

255 Jackson, M. P. and Valencia, M. 1979, *Financial aid through social work*, Routledge and Kegan Paul: in Scottish social work departments.

256 Jackson, M. *et al.* 1977, 'Social work donors', *New Society*, 3 March 1977, p. 444: survey of material aid through Scottish social work departments.

257 Jackson, M. P. *et al.* 1979, 'Variations in the provision of financial aid through social work in Scottish local authorities', *Policy and Politics*, Vol. 7, no. 1, pp. 69–81.

XII *Mental disorder and addiction*

258 Armstrong, G. *et al.* 1980, *Mentally handicapped under-fives: Leeds and Sheffield services as seen by parents*, University of Sheffield, Evaluation Research Group Report no. 8.

259 Brown, G. W. and Harris, T. 1978, *Social origins of depression: a study of psychiatric disorder in women*, Tavistock: includes population surveys in Camberwell and the Orkneys.

260 Dean, K. G. and James, H. D. 1981, 'Social factors and admission to psychiatric hospital: schizophrenia in Plymouth', *Transactions Institute of British Geographers*, new series, Vol. 6, no. 1, pp. 39–52: areal analysis.

261 Freeman, H. L. 1978, 'Mental health and the environment', *British Journal of Psychiatry*, Vol. 132, pp. 113–24: review article, of British and American literature.

262 Jones, K. *et al.* 1975, *Opening the door: a study of new policies for the mentally handicapped*, Routledge and Kegan Paul: includes a survey of practices in eleven local authority areas in Yorkshire, before reorganisation.

263 Kane, G. P. 1981, *Inner city alcoholism: an ecological analysis and cross-cultural study*, Human Sciences Press: American.

264 Kilich, S. and Plant, M. A. 1981, 'Regional variations in the levels of alcohol related problems in Britain', *British Journal of Addiction*, Vol. 76, no. 1, pp. 47–62.

265 Knight, L. 1979, 'Secure units: fact or fiction?', *Mind Out*, no. 33, pp. 10–12: 'it is almost five years since a Government circular was issued asking Regional Health Authorities to set up regional secure units. Not a single unit has yet been built, and only six RHAs have interim units. Reports on the action, or lack of it, region by region.'

266 Mind 1976, *The next step: community care for former psychiatric patients in six towns*, National Association for Mental Health.

267 Mittler, P. 1963, 'Services for the mentally subnormal', *New Society*, 17 October 1963, pp. 14–16: comparison of local authorities' provision and plans, on the occasion of Cmnd 1973.

268 Murray, J. and Knight, L. 1976, 'Ready to leave? A survey on rehabilitation and after-care for mentally ill patients', *Community Care*, 23 June 1976, pp. 16–24: survey of forty-seven mental hospitals in England and Wales, with tabulated comparison between them.

269 Rehin, G. F. and Martin, F. M. 1968, *Patterns of performance in community care: a report of a community mental health services study*, Oxford University Press: compares services in Oldham, Salford and Worthing.

270 Revans, R. W. and Baquer, A. 1972, *'I thought they were supposed to be doing that': a comparative study of co-ordination of services for the mentally handicapped in seven local authorities between June 1969 and September 1972*, King's Fund Centre.

271 Ryan, P. and Wing, J. K. 1979, 'Patterns of residential care: a study of hostels and group homes used by four local authorities to support mentally ill people in the community', in M. R. Olsen (ed.) 1979, *The care of the mentally disordered*, Birmingham, BASW: London boroughs of Camden, Islington, Newham and Redbridge.

272 Seed, P. 1981, *Mental handicap: who helps in rural and remote communities?*, Tunbridge Wells, Costello Educational: in Scotland.

273 Thompson, R. 1976, *Residential and day care services for the mentally handicapped and mentally ill in the London boroughs 1966–1974*, Greater London Council Research Memo. no. 489.

274 Webb, S. D. 1978, 'Mental health in rural and urban environments', *Ekistics*, Vol. 45, no. 266, pp. 37–42.

XIII Offenders

275 Baldwin, J. and Bottoms, A. E. 1976, *The urban criminal: a study of Sheffield*, Tavistock: empirical study compares different areas of the city.

276 Davids, X. 1969, 'Sentences for cannabis offences', *New Society*, 6 March 1969, p. 368: geographical variations in sentencing.

277 Davidson, R. N. 1981, *Crime and environment*, Croom Helm: geographical and environmental distribution of incidence of reported crime.

278 Ditchfield, J. A. 1976, *Police cautioning in England and Wales*, HMSO, Home Office Research Study no. 37: following the Children and Young Persons Act, 1969.

279 Giller, H. and Morris, A. 1977, 'Juvenile courts or children's hearings?', *Legal Action Group bulletin*, October 1977, pp. 227–9: comparing the English and Scottish systems.

280 Herbert, D. 1982, *The geography of urban crime*, Longman: 'examines the data bases for the study of crime, the theories of criminology, the areal and ecological dimensions of criminality, the patterns of offences and problem areas, and concludes with an assessment of the direction of research and policy implications'; examples from south Wales.

281 Martin, F. M. *et al.* 1981, *Children out of court*, Scottish Academic Press: children's hearings in Scotland, implications for juvenile system in the rest of Britain.

282 Martin, F. and Murray, K. (eds.) 1976, *Children's hearings*, Scottish Academic Press: in Scotland.

283 Parker, R. and Williams, B. 1976, 'Probation officers and parole supervision', *Probation Journal*, Vol. 23, no. 4, pp. 112–17: NAPO survey in three London boroughs.

284 Turner, J. 1978, 'Scotland v. England', *New Society*, 8 June 1978, pp. 539–40: compares English juvenile courts with Scottish children's hearings.

XIV Racial minorities

285 Commission for Racial Equality 1978, *Multi-racial Britain: the social services' response*, CRE: local authority social services departments are slow to take up available funds, national survey.

286 Connelly, N. 1981, *Social services provision and multi-racial areas*, Policy Studies Institute: interviews in two London boroughs, two metropolitan districts and two shire counties, not identified.

287 Cripps, J. 1977, *Accommodation for gypsies: a report on the working of the Caravan Sites Act, 1968*, HMSO.

288 Knight, L. 1976, 'Race: where were we?', *Community Care*, 21 July 1976, pp. 14–16: integration in Southall and Newham, and the social services departments' reactions.

289 Puxon, G. 1973, 'No room at the verge', *New Society*, 6 December 1973, p. 595: gypsies, and geographical inequality in implementation of the Caravan Sites Act, 1968.

290 Nixon, J. 1980, 'The importance of communication in the implementation of government policy at the local level', *Policy and Politics*, Vol. 8, no. 2, pp. 127–46: operation of the Race Relations Act, 1976 in two contrasted London boroughs.

291 Peach, C. *et al*. (eds.) 1981, *Ethnic segregation in cities*, Croom Helm.

292 Russell, F. P. Ltd. 1980, *Research results of attitudes towards the non-British population in Great Britain*, Frost Phillips Russell Ltd.: street interviews in twelve provincial centres.

XV Social work and community work services

293 Bailey, N. *et al*. 1980, *Resourcing communities: evaluating the experience of six area resource centres*, Polytechnic of Central London: EEC funded anti-poverty research.

294 Brown, A. 1978, 'Why no social worker on the Scillies?', *Community Care*, 18 January 1978, p. 3: part of the UK effectively without social work services.

295 Carver, V. and Edwards, J. L. 1972, *Social workers and their work loads*, National Institute for Social Work Training: 'the report of an investigation into work time and work patterns of 572 social work personnel employed in the health and/or welfare departments of eighteen local authorities in England and Wales for two weeks in October/November 1969 and in associated voluntary agencies.' Includes comments on differences between authorities.

296 Davies, B. and Barton, A. 1974, 'Area and authority determinants of the calibre of junior administrators', *Policy and Politics*, Vol. 3, no. 2, pp. 71–92: analysis of performance of candidates for Local Government Training Board exams., from welfare and children's departments in administrative counties and county boroughs between 1965 and 1970.

297 Deakin, R. and Willmott, P. 1979, *Participation in local social services: an exploratory study*, Personal Social Services Council: in two London borough social services department area teams.

298 Department of Health and Social Security, Social Work Service 1975, 'The service delivery study', *Social Work Service*, 6 June 1975, pp. 1–22: wide-ranging study made in 1973 of thirty-five social services departments selected, 'to include a geographical spread throughout England and Wales, with examples of urban and rural communities, high and low density populations, large and

small authorities and a variety of organisational patterns'. Individual authorities are not identified.

299 Draper, J. and Brown, A. 1978, 'The long, lonely wait on the picket lines', *Community Care*, 29 November 1978, pp. 4–5: assessing the impact of social work strikes in Southwark and Newcastle.

300 English, J. and Martin, F. M. (eds.) 1979, *Social Services in Scotland*, Scottish Academic Press: historical development.

301 Evans, R. 1979, 'Striking facts – a survey of fieldworkers', *Community Care*, 8 March 1979, pp. 16–18: social workers attitudes to the strikes, from interviews in two social services departments.

302 Kakabadse, A. 1982, *Culture of the social services*, Gower: compares twelve social services departments, management aspects.

303 Kakabadse, A. P. and Worrall, R. 1978, 'Job satisfaction and organisational structure: a comparative study of nine social services departments', *British Journal of Social Work*, Vol. 8, no. 1, pp. 51–70.

304 Kakabadse, A. 1979, 'Organisational structure and attitudes to work', *Management Decision*, Vol. 17, no. 2, pp. 189–201: in nine social services departments.

305 Parsloe, P. 1981, *Social services area teams*, George Allen and Unwin: based on DHSS funded research, see ref. 307.

306 Stevenson, O. 1978, 'Seebohm – seven years on', *New Society*, 2 February 1978, pp. 249–51: study of area teams in eight local authorities in England, Scotland and Northern Ireland; authorities not identified.

307 Stevenson, O. *et al*. 1978, *Social services teams: the practitioner's view*, HMSO: study of thirty-one area teams in eight local authorities in England, Scotland and Northern Ireland, authorities not identified; DHSS funded research.

308 Taylor, M. 1980, *Street level: two resource centres and their users*, Community Projects Foundation: Manchester and Tyne-and-Wear.

309 Waler, R. *et al*. 1972, *Social workers and their workloads in Northern Ireland welfare departments*, National Institute for Social Work Training: similar to the Carver and Edwards study in England and Wales, see ref. 295.

XVI Voluntary organisations

310 Braithwaite, G. 1974, 'South East London Consortium', *Social Work Today*, 30 May 1974, p. 135: coordinating agency for voluntary organisations in the south London boroughs.

311 Chamberlayne, P. 1976, 'The political context of community action', *Social Work Today*, 16 September 1976, p. 359: attitudes of four London boroughs to participation by local political party members, community activists and volunteers.

312 Cousins, P. F. 1976, 'Voluntary organisations and local government in three south London boroughs', *Public Administration*, Vol. 54, no. 1, pp. 63–81.

313 Harrison, P. 1973, 'The neighbourhood council', *New Society*, 12 April 1973, p. 73: how neighbourhood councils function in Liverpool, Stockport, Lambeth and North Kensington.

314 Hatch, S. and Mocroft, I. 1977, 'Factors affecting the location of voluntary organisation branches', *Policy and Politics*, Vol. 6, pp. 163–72: from the Wolfenden committee research on the incidence of local branches of some national charities.

315 Hatch, S. 1980, *Outside the state: voluntary organisations in three English*

towns, Croom Helm: incidence and characteristics of the organisations, from surveys originally done for the Wolfenden report, ref. 317.

316 Taub, R. B. *et al.* 1977, 'Urban voluntary associations: locality based and externally induced', *American Journal of Sociology*, Vol. 83, no. 2, pp. 425–42: American.

317 Wolfenden Committee 1977, *The future of voluntary organisations*, Croom Helm: chapter three includes an account of surveys undertaken in three English and one Scottish town, of the incidence and characteristics of voluntary organisations: little detail, and the towns are not identified.

Note

Place of publication for books, journals and periodicals is not given where this is available through standard sources of reference (*Publishers' international directory*, Library Association; *Directory of publishing*, Cassell & Publishers' Association; *Ulrich's international periodical directory*, Bowker; *Willing's press guide*, Thomas Skinner Directories). Pamphlets are published in London unless another town is given. In most cases the publisher of a pamphlet will be an organisation that is listed in the telephone directory for the appropriate town.

Abbreviations

ADSS	Association of Directors of Social Services
BASW	British Association of Social Workers
CES	Centre for Environmental Studies (closed)
CHAR	Campaign for the Homeless and Rootless
CIPFA	Chartered Institute of Public Finance and Accountancy
CURS	Centre for Urban and Regional Studies, University of Birmingham
DoE	Department of the Environment (UK government)
DHSS	Department of Health and Social Security (UK government)
EEC	European Economic Community
HMSO	UK government publisher
LAMSAC	Local Authorities Management Services and Computer Committee
LCSS	London Council of Social Service (renamed London Voluntary Service Council)
NAB	National Assistance Board (UK government)
NAPO	National Association of Probation Officers
n.d.	no date of publication given, a date following in brackets is a reliable guess
NISW	National Institute for Social Work
NWAF	National Women's Aid Federation
OPCS	Office of Population Censuses and Surveys (UK government)
PA	(not known)
RHA	regional health authority
SAUS	School for Advanced Urban Studies, University of Bristol
SCD	Scottish Council on Disability
SHAC	Shelter Housing Aid Centre
SOLACE	Society of Local Authority Chief Executives
SSD	social services department
WWA	Welsh Women's Aid

Index

In this index the following abbreviations are used: NHS = National Health Service; NI = Northern Ireland; Scot = Scotland.